Love, OLIVIA

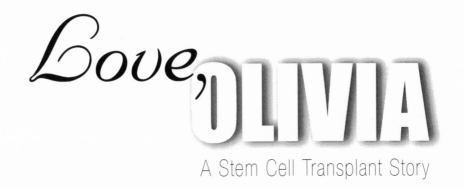

# Love, Olivia

## A Stem Cell Transplant Story

## OLIVIA CHIN *and*
## DR. TOMER MARK

WESTBOW
PRESS
A DIVISION OF THOMAS NELSON

WestBow Press books may be ordered through booksellers or by contacting:

WestBow Press
A Division of Thomas Nelson
1663 Liberty Drive
Bloomington, IN 47403
www.westbowpress.com
1-(866) 928-1240

ISBN: 978-1-4497-3554-8 (sc)
ISBN: 978-1-4497-3555-5 (hc)
ISBN: 978-1-4497-3553-1 (e)

Library of Congress Control Number: 2011963200

Printed in the United States of America

WestBow Press rev. date: 2/21/2012

*I dedicate this book to Wai, whom I love with all my heart, to Dr. Ruben Niesvizky and Dr. Tomer Mark, who are making it possible for me to spend more time hounding him, and to my mother, who has taken the brunt of my anger.*

*I hope this book helps others deal with the unexpected and will help my daughters someday understand who their mother was.*

# FOREWORD

Eleven million cancer survivors will celebrate birthdays in 2011, thanks to scientific research, early detection through screening, new therapies, advocacy, and patient support by organizations such as the American Cancer Society.

A cancer diagnosis is difficult. Having to travel away from home for treatment only adds to the level of stress experienced by patients and their family and friends. That is why over forty years ago the American Cancer Society created Hope Lodge, a place where cancer patients and their caregivers can find help while away from home. Not having to worry about where to stay or how to pay for lodging allows patients, with the support of their caregivers, to focus on getting well.

Hope Lodge NYC, located in midtown Manhattan, is one of thirty-one Hope Lodges nationwide (as of 2011). It provides lodging and support in a nurturing environment where guests can retreat to the privacy of their rooms or connect with others who *share* the cancer journey. Informational, educational, therapeutic, and social resources and information about how best to fight cancer are offered completely free of charge to its guests. The services provided by Hope Lodge complement the expert treatment patients receive at our city's world-class cancer hospitals. It is also our aim to help reduce the financial and emotional stress that often accompanies a cancer diagnosis and treatment.

While the American Cancer Society's Hope Lodge NYC is in and of itself a beautiful facility, it is its guests, the remarkable patients and their family members and friends, who make it a magical place. Their smiles, caring spirit, and determination to live are infectious and put our daily existence into great perspective. They give and receive support in this unique community of patients, caregivers, volunteers, and staff.

Olivia Chin is a wife, mother, family member, and friend. She is an extraordinary individual who at one time was a guest of our Hope Lodge NYC and who will forever remain part of our family. She traveled from her upstate New York home in Owego to New York City to receive her life-saving treatment. In writing *Love, Olivia*, she has captured her journey over a multi-year period through an unusual collection of personal e-mail exchanges. She draws us into her family life and her deepest thoughts as she fights for her life and educates us about the science behind a stem cell transplant. Medical perspectives and information are provided by her treating physician, Dr. Tomer Mark of Weill-Cornell School of Medicine.

Olivia is a soft-spoken and intelligent woman who has a "glass 100 percent full" approach to life and its inconveniences. She has an amazing sense of humor that comes through easily in both verbal and written forms. In fact, she is hysterically funny much of the time!

From diagnosis to discoveries and decisions, Olivia has had experiences that would make others give up, but she has faced them with optimism and a sense of style. She has had her share of ups and downs, but has managed to continue her journey with humor, grace, courage, and humanity, and with a smile on her beautiful face.

Olivia's story is synonymous with survivorship; it is a source of inspiration to her family, friends, the medical community, and, hopefully, to others in need. In this book, she speaks to the importance of finding answers, having a community of support, and always keeping hope alive!

Karen L. Radwin
Senior Managing Executive
American Cancer Society Hope Lodge NYC

# INTRODUCTION

Getting a diagnosis of a deadly disease is like being hit by a tractor-trailer. How we first react to this diagnosis takes us down individual paths. How we come to grips with this diagnosis often involves the support of others. How we get through treatment with this diagnosis—it takes a village. This is the story of my village.

In the fall of 2006, I had severe pain in my back and legs. Being an active mother of two young girls, I figured this pain was due to excessive hauling and schlepping, in particular because our house in upstate New York had been flooded that summer. I started with my family physician, who has known me for many years. She was familiar with my childhood collection of diseases, and she was my attending physician while I enhanced my collection as an adult. Looking back, there were definite signs of autoimmune issues.

Through 2007, we ran through test after test and scan after scan. Eventually, some blood test results gave my doctor cause for concern, and she referred me to a hematologist. The hematologist ran through more tests, the results of which determined that I had MGUS. MGUS is a condition to be monitored that may lead to cancer. The only problem was that MGUS is typically asymptomatic, which could not explain the worsening pain in my leg and foot.

I went for a second opinion in New York City at Weill-Cornell in December of 2008. After seeing two dermatologists, one chiropractor, two massage therapists, two podiatrists, one hematologist, one rheumatologist, two neurologists, one nephrologist, one blood pathologist, and one neurosurgeon, the second hematologist arrived at the diagnosis of primary AL amyloidosis (amyloid light chain). This was the equivalent of getting a death sentence. What I did not know was that the second hematologist, Dr. Ruben Niesvizky, is one of the leading experts in multiple myeloma. I am still not sure what prompted him to re-run a particular test. This was a test that had already been performed in upstate New York. Was it experience, intuition, or genius? The result indicated I had multiple myeloma and secondary amyloidosis. The treatment was a stem cell transplant. This was the equivalent to getting parole.

I had my diagnosis by late spring of 2009. Two weeks later, I went through a stem cell transplant. I had the absolute best care between Dr. Niesvizky, Dr. Tomer Mark, and their teams. Their administrative staff members, Patty and Alana, put up with a lot every day, and they still manage to deal with every situation with humor. The hospital staff at the stem cell unit at New York Presbyterian Hospital—from the cleaning lady to the nurses to the attending physicians—shall remain in my heart forever.

These people are all part of my village. The American Cancer Society Hope Lodge, NYC in Manhattan provided my first glimpse into the larger village. Being with other cancer patients made me realize that we can cope for decades with deadly cancers, beating all the odds and supporting each other with hope and love. My village includes the community of incredible friends who circled around my family like protective angels, taking my girls through an unimaginable spring and summer. My husband, Wai, rose to the occasion and was quietly and gently supportive. My brother, Nicky who lives in Nairobi, Kenya, came and played with the kids for two weeks. Friends called and sent cards and e-mails. My faith grew in leaps and bounds—not because of the disease, but in spite of it.

During this period, the economy crashed and burned. The area I live in has one major employer, and one out of four employees was laid off during this time. A retirement package became available, and we were not able to take it due to a lapse in health insurance coverage. But my village came through. Our family and friends showered us with care and love. There is always going to be someone who hurts you badly when you are down—but then there are those who lift you up. I had never asked for help for my family before, and instead took foolish pride in providing it to others. It was really hard to ask for help. But we did. Help came pouring in—overwhelming help, selfless help, loving help. We experienced a second flood—an inundation of care and concern.

After the stem cell transplant, life started up very slowly, in bits and pieces, between naps and long periods of rest and sleep. Our village was there for us. It sustained us. It helped me recover physically, but it also helped me grow mentally and spiritually.

My village has a name. I dub it Hope. Will you please come join my village?

Love,
Olivia

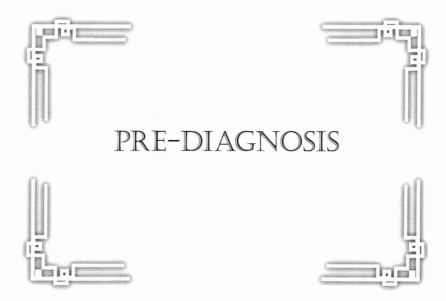

# PRE-DIAGNOSIS

From: Olivia Chin (oliviac@yahoo.com)     Sent: 12/06/2007 1:12 PM
To: "Nick You"
Cc:
Subject: Ow!

Dear Nicky,

Your little sister is in trouble.

NO, I AM NOT PREGNANT!

I have this persistent roving pain in my feet, knees, and back. I am being tested for Lyme disease, rheumatoid arthritis, lupus, and . . . gout.

Gout? I thought only salty, old seafaring sailors who drink too much have gout! Whilst there is a river in our backyard, I hardly think that qualifies us as seafaring folk. I did some reading, and gout apparently is prevalent amongst many people. I vaguely remember one of your wives having gout. Wasn't it wife number two? What remedies besides prescription drugs did she use?

Anyway, the pain is bad enough that when you come in March, you will see me hobbling about. No more high heels for me! I am reduced to what are delicately called "comfort shoes." This is a huge blow to my ego. Due to my less-than-model figure, my clothing selection has been limited to what fits (to avoid gangrene setting in from the waist down) and what hides (camouflage). However, shoes were my glory! Imelda, my hero!

Shod in scruffy slip-ons, we are busy with the day-to-day routine. Wai and the kids are fine. Katie and Elizabeth are still dancing. Both are doing very well in school. Katie is growing up into an independent person with a wicked sense of dark humor. Elizabeth just charms your socks off.

See you soon!

*Love,*
*Olivia*

# HOLIDAY NEWSLETTER 2007

It's hard for me to believe that a whole year has passed since I last sat down to write to you. We had an uneventful year—no floods, locusts, plagues, or famines! I was delighted to spend a lot of time this summer doing very little and letting the girls be girls. Our most memorable time this summer was crabbing in Long Island with our close friends—the girls screaming when hoisting the traps and seeing the scrabbling crabs!

Katie is ten. She loves to read and is interested in science and math. Elizabeth is eight. She is very social and enjoys math too. Both girls are still dancing. They danced in their first *Nutcracker* ballet this year and had a great time being mice, flowers, and snowflakes. They are preparing again for dance competitions now. Katie is headstrong, intelligent, and independent. She brings to mind a young sapling with a strong, solid trunk. Her room is neat, organized, and everything has its place. She chose several dark wood antique pieces for her room; it looks very traditional. I think it rather reflects her. Elizabeth is a charmer. She brings to mind a luxurious tall grass that sways with the wind and sashays with the music of the earth. Her room is a-flit with butterflies . . . when you can see them. I have been known to look in her room and scream in horror at the state of total chaos. What her room reflects I do not know and do not want to know.

My mother is doing well. She continues to slow down. Like a grand old tree in winter, her energy retreats in order to see spring. We went to Switzerland this summer to enjoy time together, to weave a tapestry of three generations, to create memories for the girls.

Wai is busier than ever at work. At home, his basement workshop is gone due to the flood last summer, as are the sounds of tools and the smell of freshly cut wood that used to waft up from below. He is trying to make some sense of the basement; it is a long, arduous task. Speaking of which, this was the year that marked our twenty-fifth wedding anniversary. If it were possible to tell your younger self what you know now, what would you say? If the tapestry of life were to fold upon itself, what would you want to know from your future? I would tell my younger self to say "I do" all over again and to grow together, enriching each other, not diminishing. I would say that over a lifetime together there will be times when one has to prove oneself over and over, times of knowing one has found one's soul mate, times building the Great Wall of Doubt as to whether anyone should ever come that close to you again, and times knowing there isn't a single thing you would change. There will be times for the fantasy of flight and times when you know you are filling your destiny in this lifetime.

One the lighter side—did you know we have had royal titles in our family for several years? We have Princess Frozen Peas (Katie), Princess Split Pea (Elizabeth), Queen Sweet Pea (guess who?), and our very own King Legume (Wai). Elizabeth came home from school indignant over a correction from her teacher; she had submitted a paper where she had written "human bean." She firmly believed she was right. Once home, she got very upset when we told her she was wrong. She maintained that we always told her that we were human beans . . . years of therapy . . .

May this holiday season find you in good health and spirits!

*Love,*
*Olivia*

From: Olivia Chin (oliviac@yahoo.com)    Sent: 03/18/2008 9:32 AM
To: "Nick You"
Cc:
Subject: Beer inventory way down

Dear Nicky,

It was great seeing you. Thank you for all of your help at the benefit for the Navy helicopter pilot that I was asked to organize. I thought you did a great job dishing out salad all day. I now realize you were strategically placed near the beer tap. Our community raised over $17K for the pilot and his family. I cannot imagine the impact of his sudden loss of mobility. I felt really proud of what we did. I am glad you were in town to see what your sister does for fun. You met some of my friends who organize fundraisers and benefits. And we are balloon artists—all in our spare time.

Not much else is new. I started volunteering as a middle school technology teacher at the school Katie and Elizabeth attend. It's a little hard because there is more walking than I realized—going from student to student at their laptops. I am learning to take extra painkillers before each session. They are creating a two—sided threefold brochure, so they are learning about columns, editing, importing text, and graphics, as well as how to present information. It has also been interesting observing the children in Katie's class. Elizabeth is still in elementary school. Middle school starts in fifth grade here and runs through eighth grade. I think kids mutate during middle school.

It feels good to be with these kids, even though some of them are mouthy. I gave up coaching Odyssey of the Mind this year because physically I knew I couldn't handle it.

Mom is doing alright this winter. I take her grocery shopping, and we have lunch together every now and then. It's a weird situation—I feel she lives her life through ours, and I wish there was some way to have her be involved with other people. But at eighty-nine years of age, perhaps it's just too hard to make new friends.

Love,
Olivia

From: Olivia Chin (oliviac@yahoo.com)     Sent: 04/04/2008 8:43 PM
To: "Nick You"
Cc:
Subject: Mom Hurt

Dear Nicky,

Just a very quick note.

Mom had a leg cramp yesterday morning, and she decided to get out of bed to put weight on her leg. She ended up falling and hurt herself. She fractured vertebrae. She is in a lot of pain. So far we've been to the doctor, to x-ray, and back to the doctor. A hospital bed is being delivered to her house tomorrow morning. We will set it up in her dining room.

She is mobile, and she is alright by herself. I made sure she has food in the house that she can heat up in the microwave, and we talk on the phone every morning and every evening. I stop by once a day. It hurts her to get up and open the door, so she asked me to just unlock the door and let myself in.

All is well with us. I have been to doctors a lot lately too. When pain hits suddenly, as with mom, you have to adjust in a drastic way to accommodate what you can no longer do. In my case, I just realized my life has changed significantly although ever so subtly to deal with the ever-growing pain. The ache feels like it is inside my bones.

The two of us are both popping painkillers like candy!

*Love,*
*Olivia*

From: Olivia Chin (oliviac@yahoo.com)    Sent: 04/08/2008 9:22 PM
To: "Nick You"; "Felicia"
Cc:
Subject: Glowing in the Dark

Dear Felicia and Nicky,

I am relying on you to be with me, physically, spiritually, and intellectually.

Felicia, you don't know what I am talking about, so here goes ... Last year
was a rapid descent into hell in terms of pain in my feet and joints. After
eliminating a lot of possibilities, I ended up going to a hematologist three
days ago. Since this Tuesday, I have been pricked, poked, and radiated.
We're talking CT scans, X-rays, blood tests, and urine samples. Yet to
come are the bone and bone marrow samples to be taken next week
(ow!). We've ruled out rheumatoid arthritis, gout, syphilis, Lyme disease,
and lupus. My family physician even ran a thorough blood test for food
and environmental allergies. I am allergic to dust mites and their poop.
It's a good thing we just got a cleaning lady, since I wasn't able to handle
the vacuum anymore. She got rid of some dust bunnies that we were
beginning to think of as pets and probably several million dust mites.
And their poop.

The bad news is that it might be lymphoma or myeloma. The good
news is that it might be some other disease—but I've been told if it is
something else, it's still nothing I want. The blood markers are pointing
to bone marrow issues. The latest data:

Sed rate        69
IgG total       2637
Total protein   8.1

We should know within two weeks—the results of the bone and marrow
tests should either indicate or rule out lymphoma or myeloma.

To top it all off, I got the phone call to see the hematologist while
taking mom for X-rays. She fractured vertebrae. Between taking her
to doctors, getting her appointments straightened out, dealing with her

insurance, the hospital bed, and taking care of a sick child, I had all of fifteen minutes to think about what it meant to see a hematologist in *oncology*. The receptionist who scheduled the appointment for me with the hematologist tried very hard to give me directions to his office without saying he also practices oncology!

This is how I have decided to deal with whatever is coming:

1) I am only doing those things which I have to do . . . AND
2) I am only doing that which gives me great joy . . . AND
3) I am getting rid of those people in my life who suck life out of me—we all know certain people who walk into a room, and the lights dim ever so slightly.

I have also realized that I really have little to no control over whatever is coming next. I cannot will test results. I cannot make numbers change. I cannot alter biopsy results. So I am going to exercise control over what I can: my attitude. I can sit and mope during the day and moan in the moonlight, or I can try to laugh through whatever comes.

I choose laughter.

I have the first good news since my whole saga started—the full body X-rays (all nineteen of them) showed no lesions. (After this week, I now glow in the dark. If you look very, very carefully, there are even blinking lights!)

Love,
Olivia

From: Olivia Chin (oliviac@yahoo.com)    Sent: 04/17/2008 6:18 AM
To: "Nick You"
Cc:
Subject: Squeeze, Scream, and Bite

Dear Nicky,

I had the bone sample and bone marrow sample taken out yesterday. Not fun. Then there were two more CT scans and about twenty-six X-rays since Tuesday. I should have a diagnosis for lymphoma or myeloma soon. I am still hoping it could be something else, preferably less deadly. I got the results of the scans today. There are still no bone lesions, so that is good news.

I need to tell Mom soon, assuming a diagnosis will be made. If it is not lymphoma or myeloma, the search starts all over again. If it is lymphoma or myeloma, be prepared for me to ask you for help. What is your work schedule? I think it would be better for Mom to have you near after I tell her.

Here's hoping it's something else . . . or at least in a smoldering stage. (The terminology is smoldering or active).

Hey—I got the nurse to give me chocolate during the bone marrow sampling. She asked me if I was a squeezer or a screamer. I told her I was all that and also a biter, but when given chocolate, I cease to bite. Since it was her job to let me squeeze her, and the position I was in meant her hands were next to my mouth, she got me chocolate, pronto!

The doctor had a really hard time. He says I have hard, solid bones. He struggled to get to the marrow. When he asked if I work out, he had to ask me to stop laughing because I was jiggling from giggling so much. After several tries, I asked him if it was possible if my bones were not that hard but that perhaps he had lost his muscle tone. This is not a good question to ask your doctor when he has a metal tube going through your rump into your bone. Not good at all.

There is no dignity.

Love,
Olivia

From: Nick You  Sent: 04/19/2008 3:02 PM
To: "Olivia Chin"
Cc:
Subject: RE: Squeeze, Scream, and Bite

Dear Olivia,

Walked by a church today, went in, and lit a candle for you. Stubborn bones ... Runs in the family. Am free all of August, busy before, and have a very important mission second week of November. That's it.

Nicky

From: Olivia Chin (oliviac@yahoo.com)     Sent: 04/21/2008 9:07 PM
To: "Nick You"
Cc:
Subject: RE: Squeeze, Scream, and Bite

Dear Nicky,

Just keep the candle burning within.

Hey—stop being so morose. Consider the following that I survived:

Whooping cough
Eye surgeries
Tonsils the size of tennis balls (obviously removed)
Viral meningitis
Hepatitis A
TB
Double DVTs
Complete hysterectomy
Strep that went septic

        AND

Twenty-six years of marriage to Wai.

So what makes you think I won't lick this?

*Love,*
*Olivia*

PS: Every time I go to a new doctor and fill out the medical history report, they look at me funny.

From: Olivia Chin (oliviac@yahoo.com)    Sent: 07/12/2008 8:42 PM
To: "Nick You"; "Felicia"
Cc:
Subject: Woof

Dear Felicia and Nicky,

My calendar is filled with all these meetings with rich men. Too bad they are all doctors.

I have been to a podiatrist who gave me a shot in the ankle with a syringe that I thought only veterinarians used on large farm animals. I wanted to bite him on the leg.

I have been to a rheumatologist who examined me and, while checking out my joints, made my foot go instantly numb. It has stayed numb, much to my dismay. The numbness has been joined by the sensation of pins and needles now. I almost bit him on the arm.

I have been to a dermatologist who was an absolute waste of time and told me that I just needed to put cream on the rash that is all over my body. I tried to bite her finger.

I have been to a kidney specialist who said I was getting close to aspirin toxicity, considering how many I have been taking. So we are off aspirin and on acetaminophen, which doesn't work as well for me. I now want to bite anyone close to me.

I have been to my family physician so often that I am thinking about asking for a dedicated chair in her waiting room far away from other chairs so I don't bite other patients waiting there.

I think I will come back as a dog in another life.

Love,
Olivia

# PRE-DIAGNOSIS:
# MEDICAL PERSPECTIVE

The time that a person must wait between realizing that there is something wrong with their bodies or their health and learning what exactly that something can be fills him or her with anything from mere uncertainty to complete terror. What Olivia first experienced was a gradually increasing painful sensation in her feet. Foot pain is common in the general public, and when she first went to see her family doctor, she naturally started looking for common causes. One of the first lessons of medical training is that you are much more likely to see an unusual presentation of a common disease rather than a textbook presentation of a rare disease; in other words, when you hear hoof beats, think horses—not zebras. Her doctor started by doing the right thing and trying to rule out common things first.

The pain that Olivia had in her feet could be the presentation for a number of different ailments. To name a few possibilities: arthritis, tendonitis, gout, rheumatoid arthritis, peripheral neuropathy, lyme disease, etc. A battery of tests were performed to look for these conditions first in Olivia. What made her doctors probe deeper, however, was the elevation of a protein called a monoclonal protein, also known as a M-spike, M-protein, or paraprotein.

The M-protein is a by-product of a clonal dysregulation in immune function. A healthy immune system can be thought of as a team of many different players, each with a specific job. Some cells respond to bacterial infections, others secrete factors that bind to and inhibit parasites, and still others act to direct other cells in a series of complex interactions between the body and a foreign invader, such as rhinovirus (aka. the common cold).

One of the most basic divisions in terms of immune function is that between innate and humoral immunity. The innate immune system is the evolutionarily older branch; components of the immune system are designed to directly recognize and destroy targets that could be harmful for the body. For instance, the job of a specific type of cell called the neutrophil is to hunt around the body and gobble up bacteria by secreting enzymes. Humoral immunity can be found in sharks and higher vertebrates. Humoral immunity exists to direct and amplify the innate immune response, giving the benefit of a focused burst of immune activity and also leading to immunologic memory. The major cellular components of humoral immunity are T and B cells. These cells establish the memory that you had chicken pox as a child and serve to prevent infection upon future re-exposure.

T and B cells are further broken down into smaller subsets. While we won't get into the details here, one that deserves highlighting is the *plasma cell*. The plasma cell is the most mature (or differentiated) type of B cell. This cell is responsible for the production and secretion of antibodies. Antibodies (also called immunoglobulins) are proteins that that are designed to stick to parts of bacteria, viruses, fungi, and other things that could potentially make your body sick. When an antibody finds and is bound to its target (called an antigen), your body knows that something is amiss and quickly goes into action (either by getting rid of the antibody-antigen complex directly or by stimulating the innate immune system) to bring it back to the status quo. When we get an infection, antibodies of all shapes and sizes, corresponding to different antigens, rise in our bloodstream. The plasma cells that generate the antibodies that happen to be specific for the current infection become very active, producing large amounts of immunoglobulin and growing in number. When the infection clears, the plasma cells fall back into a resting state and the antibody levels in the blood fall.

An M-protein arises when the plasma cell doesn't follow the rules described above. An M-protein represents a single (hence the "mono"clonal) type of antibody that undergoes continued production by a group of plasma cells. These plasma cells are thought to be all derived from one single miscreant progenitor. Sometimes, all the plasma cells do is stay in a small pack, make a small amount of M-protein, and then call it a day. This situation is very common; the medical term for it is **Monoclonal Gammopathy of Undetermined Significance (MGUS)**. The plasma cells in MGUS generally leave the body alone and the amount of M-protein is small. Most people do not know that they have MGUS, which is a good thing, since it is estimated 5-6 percent of the entire population of the United States over the age of sixty have it.

By definition, MGUS is a benign condition, usually picked up on blood work that was done to screen for other conditions (the most common pickup is when a total protein level is high on a standard chemistry blood panel). MGUS requires no treatment, since there is no manifestation of any problem in the body due to the M-protein to begin with. There is a catch though—with MGUS comes a yearly risk of progression to either lymphoma or myeloma. The risk is small—about 1-2 percent per year—but this bears at least yearly monitoring in the hematologist's office with repeat blood work.

As persons age, clonal disregulation in the immune system becomes more common. In other words, more opportunities for plasma cell dysfunction are created as time goes by, leading to more plasma cell clones. Thus, as people age, the chance of finding MGUS becomes more common. In one large study looking at banked samples of blood in the general population of Rochester, Minnesota, 3 percent of the population over sixty-five had a monoclonal protein in the blood. In people eighty-five years and older, the percentage was 7 percent.

People with MGUS should be followed by a hematologist regularly, but with the proper perspective, the level of anxiety this diagnosis induces should be low.

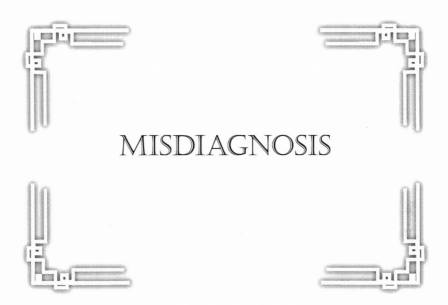

# MISDIAGNOSIS

Dear Friends,

I am sending a mass e-mail to all of you who have been wondering how I am doing. I hope you do not mind. It is easier for me than calling everyone back or responding to individual e-mails. I have been running from doctor to doctor, test to test, and my calendar overrunneth. If you do not wish to receive e-mails such as this one, please just let me know, and I will remove you from my "OHS★★T" distribution list.

I have good news! There are no lesions, no tumors, and the bone marrow looks good! The hematologist said yesterday he was convinced it was multiple myeloma last week due to the pain level and inflammation in my bones and joints. He was delighted to tell me it is currently benign.

*Thank God!*

I am in what they call the "smoldering stage" of myeloma—beyond precancerous, but not yet cancer. It is also known as MGUS (monoclonal gammopathy of undetermined significance). MGUS is a precancerous condition which has a 1 in 100 chance of turning into multiple myeloma for every year that you have it. MGUS is a term used to describe the finding of a monoclonal protein in the blood. This means an immunoglobulin keeps replicating itself and producing clones of itself. The immunoglobulins' role in the body is to attack and destroy nasty stuff that causes infections. We have several different types of good immunoglobulins. With MGUS, one of these immunoglobulins goes crazy and starts multiplying, so there is an elevation of one type, in my case IgG. We all need a balanced set of immunoglobulins to maintain an effective immune system. When one immunoglobulin type gets out of control, the balance is upset and causes the immune system to weaken. The overproduced immunoglobulin is useless at fighting infection because it is not directed at a foreign invader like a bacterium or virus. Multiple myeloma is a cancer of the plasma cells and therefore the bone marrow, as this is where plasma cells are made within the body. Beyond pain, frequent infections are a sign of the progression from MGUS to (multiple) myeloma.

*Have you noticed this is the first time I have used the word cancer?*

In my case, I was told it was probably not in the earliest stages, although that is actually unknown at this point. MGUS does not usually have any symptoms, so the question now is why I have all the pain typically associated with myeloma. The symptoms are more advanced than the lab tests. In fact, the doctor was wondering if I was blessed (blessed???) in the sense that perhaps a second underlying condition is adding to the pain, which started my search early. Also, the plan to get a second opinion from a myeloma expert is in the works. MGUS is monitored via blood tests, and goodness is when the amount of the high protein stays stable or grows at a slow rate. If the levels of the high protein keep rising, the MGUS is not stable and may mean that the condition is progressing toward myeloma. Since I just established the baseline of these proteins this week, future blood tests will be taken at regular intervals to monitor any transition of MGUS.

*I was praying that it would be MGUS. I really didn't want to lose the little hair I have left.*

There is no treatment yet. There might be some trials and experimental meds. So for now, I am being monitored while in the smoldering stage. I am feeling so lucky—this is infinitely better than having active myeloma for a period of time. Last week, the doctor discussed stem cell treatments. Yesterday, he was glad that it was MGUS, not myeloma. He joked that his only regret was that we would not see each other as much as if it were active. I let him know that I, on the hand, had absolutely no such regrets. What a relief! I saw him for the first time last Tuesday; by this Thursday, I had the CT scans, the X-rays, the bone and bone marrow samples, and the blood tests all done. By Monday morning, all results were in. I have been on the Internet looking up alternative treatments, and all I came up with is consuming turmeric.

*Indian curry—in a hurry.*

I am so blessed to have you in my life, to have so many people around me who have showered me with concern, and that so many of you have volunteered to have your bone marrow checked for matches. FYI: It wasn't that bad. The short pain was more than having a filling in a tooth, less than a root canal, and the soreness only lasted two days. The world is still a good place, filled with good people. Yesterday, I had my teeth cleaned. The dentist moved my appointment up in case chemo would start, and the two dental hygienists came to say they want to be tested for bone marrow matches. Another person I know is the wife of a Russian Orthodox priest, who is a talented Byzantine icon painter. She said her husband prayed at mass this Sunday for me, and then she gave me a traveling curing icon, saying it has always cured everyone it has touched, and to return it only after it did its magic. To each and every one of you—thanks from the heart.

*Want to buy a miraculous icon for cheap?*

It may come to chemo and stem cell someday, but for now, I'll take benign-ness one day at a time. I understand my favorite foods are now good for me (cheese, dark chocolate, and red wine), so indulgence now is guilt-free. I think a trip to Switzerland is in order! Anybody want to go? Right around now, the grapes are beginning their fermentation (moût), and I think by the end of the year, the first of the 2008 vintage will be ready!

I will keep you posted as events come up or don't. Thank you for your prayers and care. I know they work. You know I will research this thing to the end, so feel free to share my contact info with anyone you hear that is being checked out for MGUS or myeloma.

Les truffes, le vin, le pain, le Boursin . . . c'est divin! (Taken from an old ad for Boursin cheese many years ago, and modified means: "Truffles, wine, bread, Boursin cheese—divine!")

*Love,*
*Olivia*

From: Olivia Chin (oliviac@yahoo.com)    Sent: 09/11/2008 8:28 AM
To: "Nick You"; "Felicia"
Cc:
Subject: Spooky Icon

Dear Felicia and Nicky,

Something very strange has been happening that I need to share. It's hard to believe and even harder to write about. A friend of mine, Nataliya, paints icons in the Byzantine tradition. When she heard I was in pain, she brought an icon she had painted to me, covered in flannel. Upon unveiling it, I was struck by the beauty of the icon, the workmanship in the painting, the etching in the gold leaf. The icon depicts Mother Mary holding Jesus as a young child or an infant.

My friend told me that this icon has cured every person it has touched, and it travels from one afflicted person to another. She insisted that I hang it near my bed and that I pray to it often. She suggested I light candles to Mary and Jesus. To be truthful, I was very appreciative of her care, but I wasn't sure about the properties of the icon. I did put it in my bedroom downstairs. I moved there after going upstairs was too difficult.

About two days after I put the icon in my room, I woke up in the wee hours of the morning, sensing a presence in my room. Sometimes Elizabeth wakes up and comes downstairs for comfort. She comes to my bedside and stares at me intently whilst I snore in my sweet slumber until I wake hyperventilating, frightened out of my wits. So I called her name; there was no reply. Sometimes our dog, Mambo, gets out of his night area and comes to investigate those restricted areas when he thinks he is unsupervised. He even retracts his nails so as to avoid detection! So I called for Mambo; there was no quick retreat. I went back to sleep.

The next night, the same sensation of someone staring at me wakens me from my sleep. There is no insomniac daughter. There is no rove dog. Sweet slumber aside, I am slightly spooked. The next night, I leave the light on when I go to bed. The feeling of being watched awakens me again. This time, I silence my frightened breathing and concentrate on the origin of the feeling of being watched. It's the icon!

Early the next morning, I call Nataliya and tell her that her icon is spooking me out! She says that being watched is nothing—others have felt the breath of Mary emanating from the icon.

I am sleeping with the lights on now.

Love,
Olivia

From: Olivia Chin (oliviac@yahoo.com)    Sent: 11/21/2008 1:02 AM
To: "Nick You"
Cc:
Subject: Vacation

Dear Nicky,

Just a quick note to let you know we are going to Florida for two weeks.

Tonight, shortly after dinner, my family physician called and asked me to go directly to the ER. She had received some test results and said she would not be able to sleep well unless a Doppler ultrasound was done. She was worried about deep vein thrombosis (DVT). She said the ER triage nurse was waiting for me.

So off I went, stopping by to get an extra-large, super-tall venti coffee on the way. Wai said with a grin, "See you tomorrow morning!" Our experience with any ER has always been extended times spent in the waiting room. I get there, and they are waiting for me! There is no wait—I do not even get to grace a chair with my derrière. My physician, Dr. R, is on her way to the hospital! Wow! She tells me there is no DVT. I call Wai to gloat.

Once back home, my darling husband tells me he panicked. He booked all four of us for two weeks in Orlando over Thanksgiving break. With great sensitivity, he tells me he did so because he was afraid we might not be able to have a family vacation for awhile.

He may not live 'til morning.

Love,
Olivia

# HOLIDAY NEWSLETTER 2008

What a year it has been! Some years flow by like a lazy river ride, floating where the slow-moving current takes you. Others are like flume rides, with one unexpected sharp turn after another—you have no choice but to hang on in a cold, wet sweat until it is over. This year was a ride that started like a lazy river, and then somehow morphed into one of those high-tech, spinning, fast-moving rides where you scream all the way! (Can you tell we just came back from two weeks in Orlando?)

This spring (a.k.a. dance competition season), Katie and Elizabeth danced team routines, and their team received awards and trophies. Elizabeth performed her first solo; she received the highest award for her age group. When this was announced to the dancers, they did not really listen. They were too busy tapping Elizabeth's trophy cup; so very impressed with the metallic ping. The cup was made of metal—not plastic!

At the end of the school year, Katie received some middle school awards. Also on this day, the departing principal performed his Happy Feet dance for us, since he has watched my first-day-of-school boogie dance every fall. Then we had a great time with friends in Long Island—a rite of the start of summer vacation. The rest of the summer was spent mostly at home. We swam, we read, we napped.

Katie is eleven; she loves to read and is interested in science and math. Elizabeth is nine and enjoys math too. Both decided to concentrate their extracurricular efforts solely on dance this year. They danced the *Baba Yaga* ballet this year as mushrooms and Russian boys, and they were understudies for skeletons. The skeleton role has such wonderful choreography that our girls harbored hidden hopes that a skeleton dancer would . . . catch a cold . . . or . . . have car trouble on the way to the performance.

My mother is doing well. She hurt herself this fall but has mostly recovered. Wai is doing fine. For our twenty-sixth wedding anniversary, we went to Howe Caverns, where Wai and I went once before we even started dating. We noticed that some of the stalactites have grown a fraction of a millimeter since our last visit! I've been very achy this year, so I've been grumpier than usual (just imagine!). This fall, I was diagnosed with a blood disorder, and we are dealing with that just fine. I've reduced my volunteer efforts and am only doing that which is necessary, and that which gives me great joy. Good friends also give great joy. Wine and dark chocolate are also quite good. This is an approach I should have developed years ago! I recommend it highly.

My faith also continues to grow. My faith has been very rational, very intellectual. Then some inexplicable events happened with an icon and then again while with an orthodox priest. The true "leap of faith" happened this year. I've accepted that faith means believing in what you cannot prove or rationalize or touch. Like the Space Mountain ride, you have to just accept the power of the great divine full-speed in the dark!

One of the efforts that provided great joy was decorating a room in a *Nutcracker* theme in the Roberson Mansion in Binghamton for Christmas with close friends. We had a large room in the mansion to decorate for the Rafael Grigorian Ballet Theatre, a not-for-profit group that puts on productions such as *The Russian Nutcracker* and *Baba Yaga*. Other joys include making jewelry and playing with balloons. I had an exhibit of balloons for Thanksgiving at the Tioga County Council of the Arts, consisting of a cornucopia over-spilling with fruit, a turkey, a pumpkin, a wreath, a giant flower, and a framed portrait of a wacky blonde complete with pearls and a grey hair, all done with balloons. Fun with latex! Years of therapy . . .

May you all have a wonderful holiday season. Enjoy the time you have with as much spirit and fire as possible. May this holiday season find you in good health and spirits!

*Love,*
*Olivia*

From: Olivia Chin (oliviac@yahoo.com)     Sent: 01/04/2009 3:00 PM
To: Friendlist
Cc:
Subject: Happy New Year!

Dear Friends,

First of all, Happy New Year, everybody! I hope you had a good Christmas/
Hanukkah/Kwanzaa. We had a restful time a home . . . did very little . . .
ate quite a lot . . . slept in . . . napped . . . . Anyway, here is the requested
update about me.

Late last year, I had first been told to get ready for chemo and a bone
marrow transplant, only to find out two weeks later that my bone marrow
aspirate and bone sample were clean. This means no chemo and no stem
cell transplant—yet. Since then, I have been on a rampage, supporting the
medical community of Broome and Tioga counties. I have been MRI'd
thrice, CT'd twice, and I've had enough X-rays to compete with our
Christmas tree lights. I've been to podiatrists, oncologists, dermatologists,
physical therapists, nephrologists, chiropractors, and more are yet to
come.

So where am I at?

The diagnosis is currently downgraded to MGUS, with the only
outstanding unknown being the pain in the right foot and leg. An analogy
to the last fourteen months would be: You set out to shop for bread, milk,
and eggs. On the way to the market, somehow you made a detour and
bought a new car. Then you took a road trip for several months in the
new car. You finally get back home, where there is nothing to eat. So you
go to the market and purchase a delicious-looking roast, fresh vegetables,
salad, and fruit. Once home, you realize you forgot to buy bread, milk,
and eggs.

I went to find out why my foot and leg hurt. I came home with MGUS,
and I still have pain in the foot and leg. At this point, I've been told there
are three possibilities: a bunch of nerves are being pinched together in
my back by the spine or a disc; the same bunch is being pinched together

by a lesion or growth; or I have a rare form of myeloma, consisting of a localized growth around or in the leg. The only test left is a PET scan, which is waiting insurance approval. It was turned down by our 2008 insurance company, but we are switching in 2009 to another company, so it should be covered. It was turned down on Christmas Eve after having been approved. I was in the mall doing some last minute Christmas shopping when the insurance company called, and I just broke down and cried. The insurance company got myeloma and melanoma mixed up—how pathetic is that?

In December, I went to The Center for Myeloma at Weill-Cornell Medical in NYC with my friend Mary. The physician, Dr. Niesvizky, was very knowledgeable, very competent, and down-to-earth. He was able to answer all the questions I had that remained, until then, unanswered. His manner and knowledge impressed me and generated deep respect. The highlights of the trip were the physician, pastrami, and dim sum. May I say that the 2nd Avenue Deli pastrami beat out Katz's Delicatessen for us, but Katz's pickles were far superior.

I was also informed that turmeric was undergoing a clinical trial for myeloma. So we are having curry chicken, curry chickpeas, curry beef, curry meat patties, turmeric in the chili, turmeric in the rice, mustard in the sandwich, mustard in the sauce . . . If you come over and the salad looks suspiciously yellow, don't ask.

In the meantime, I was taking medication that helped a lot with the pain (the leg and foot, remember?), but then I was told to stop. My kidneys are beginning to dump protein, which is a bad thing. There are a number of reasons, one being MGUS, but the only factor we can control is eliminating the non-steroid anti-inflammation drugs (NSAIDs). Gosh darn! The era of miracle drugs is over! The pain is back with a vengeance. This means, I am meaner than ever. By early afternoon, I just feel like biting people. So unless you want to be bitten or beheaded, beware the late afternoon! By early evening, I have either sprouted fangs or have fallen asleep. So if you haven't seen me recently, it's because my social calendar has been very full with cute doctors. When things get really bad, I just fall asleep. Consistent, severe pain is not only fang-forming, but it also tires me out. I will be going back to Cornell medical for a follow-up . . . so more to come on pastrami! (Let's see, there's the Stage, the Carnegie—so many delis!).

Lastly, a lot has happened on the spiritual side. Personal growth, life lessons, the leap of faith, and having incredible things happen that one cannot explain, rationalize, or even truly understand. And this happened *before* the turmeric! So, all in all, I wouldn't change a thing. The positives far outweigh the negatives. I have found deep comfort and am awed by the powers around us. So my attitude to the whole shebang, pain, MGUS, spirituality is: Just lucky, I guess!

Wishing you a great 2009!

*Love,*
*Olivia*

PS. There seems to be many references to food . . . hmm . . .

From: Olivia Chin (oliviac@yahoo.com)   Sent: 01/08/2009 11:10 AM
To: "Nick You"
Cc:
Subject: 12 Degrees below Zero

Dear Nicky,

It is cold. My feet are cold. My nose is cold. My hands are cold. I schlep
wood to the woodstove all day and all night. I leave the ashes for Wai to
clean up.

This is rather odd. I have always had hot sweaty hands and feet. Do you
remember when we used to ski, and I never wore gloves?

On top of everything else, I had to have a root canal. Can you believe it?
What did I do wrong in a previous life?

You asked me what I found out with Dr. Niesvizky—attached are my
notes from the visit last month.

*Love,*
*Olivia*

Attachment: Q&A with Dr. Niesvizky

1)  What tests are used to determine MGUS and its progression?
    What is the accuracy of these tests?

    There are three tests used to determine progression of disease,
    which are based on protein types and levels:
    • Immunofixation: a qualitative test, it determines whether
      proteins are monoclonal or polyclonal, lambda type, and
      protein type, such as IgA, IgG, and IgM.
    • Quantitative immunoglobulins: levels of IgA, IgG, and IgM,
      and it is used for trend analysis.

- Protein electrophoresis: this provides the amount of a specific protein (immunoglobulin), also referred to as M-spike.

Accuracy is typically not an issue provided the same equipment is used for the first two tests. The third is dependent on the reading by a diagnostician. We need to monitor your free light chains and will run the urine test using a twenty-four-hour collection and thyroid test.

2) My IgG went from 1,637 to 2,364 in one month. Is this typical, atypical? What is the significance of this increase?

IgG levels can vary. You want to look at your M-spike for trend analysis. A diagnosis of multiple myeloma is made if it is over three grams per deciliter. We also follow free light chain levels (kappa and lambda) and the K:$\lambda$ ratio. The prognosis is worse if IgA and IgM levels are detected rather than if the IgG level is high.

3) What is the accuracy of the bone marrow and bone sample tests? How much depends on the location of aspiration? Can this vary a lot?

Bone marrow and bone sample test results can vary a lot by site. The result of 4 percent indicates MGUS. When this result exceeds 10 percent, we consider it multiple myeloma. The result is also subject to reader variability.

4) I've been told to take blood pressure medication to protect my kidneys, to get off acetaminophen and Meloxicam. What do you think? What pain medication do you recommend? I am also taking two drugs for diabetes. Do you have any issues with these?

Acetaminophen is all right, as is the blood pressure medication. Reduce the use of aspirin as well as any other NSAIDs. If the pain is intolerable, we use steroids, regardless of blood sugar. We also use narcotics. The order is acetaminophen, steroids, and narcotics. The alternative of insulin should be considered.

5) I have rashes all over my torso and blisters all over my fingers. Is this related to MGUS?
See Dr. W, dermatologist. We can rule out shingles.

6) I have intense soreness in my joints and bones, especially my feet and legs. Is this related to MGUS?

Pain in the bones and joints due to diabetes and myeloma are typically bilateral, meaning the pain will show up on the left and right sides. We need to determine if the pain is peripheral neuropathy and its source. See Dr. L., neurologist. In the meantime, get an MRI for the entire spine, not just lumbar only.

7) What opinion do you have on alternative or holistic remedies? How about recommendations in terms of changes to diet?

Feel free to use acupuncture, yoga, tai chi, aromatherapy, massage, and prayer. There is currently a clinical trial on the use of turmeric. You can try turmeric. We recommend avoiding certain "funky" teas touted to ward off cancer.

8) I have a very close friend of thirty years, diagnosed with multiple myeloma at about the same time as my diagnosis with MGUS. We live less than ten miles apart. We are wondering if there is an environmental factor. What do you think?

Causes of MGUS and myeloma are suspected to be hereditary and environmental. In the case of the latter, there are known clusters. Hair dye is also known to be implicated, typically not through casual use. What is the ethnic background of your friend? Greeks, Italians, and Spaniards have higher incidences of MGUS and myeloma, as do African Americans. Asian females are rare.

9) I had my hair tested. It has been falling out. They found lead in my hair. Based on where the lead showed up, the timing of exposure to lead seems to coincide with the major flood we had in our area about eighteen months ago. Do you think there is a connection between the lead and MGUS?

I have no opinion on lead.

10) Given the diagnosis of MGUS, should I have stem cells harvested now? Do I need to worry about donor match? I have only one brother who lives in Kenya. How about blood?

There is no need to harvest stem cells yet. Those of your brother are not needed. Typically, we perform autologous stem cell transplants, where you use your own stem cells. There is no need to harvest blood.

11) Besides hair loss, I am also sleeping much more than usual. I have always slept four to five hours. Now I need eight to ten hours a night. What do you think?

We will check your thyroid.

12) What recommendations do you have for me in general?

Get the blood sugar under control.

13) What clinical trials are being run?

The only clinical trial being run on MGUS patients is the aforementioned turmeric. There are a number of clinical trials being run on multiple myeloma patients.

From: Olivia Chin (oliviac@yahoo.com)     Sent: 01/18/2009 7:58 AM
To: "Nick You"; "Felicia"
Cc:
Subject: B******t

Dear Felicia and Nicky,

I am catching up from the holidays. At our house, Christmas involves cooking, baking, decorating, wrapping, tree chopping, shopping, and trying very hard to remember the main reason for the season.

After seeing the local hematologist, rheumatologist, and podiatrist, I was still concerned about the pain in my right leg and foot, and nobody had any answers. I was not able to walk much and was beginning to use a scooter. So I asked my friend Lisette, who audits clinical trials, for a recommendation. Even though I had a referral from the local hematologist to an excellent myeloma doctor for a second opinion, Lisette was sent on a quest to find a myeloma physician who was highly respected by nurses. She came up with the Multiple Myeloma Clinic at Weill-Cornell Medical in NYC. I had an appointment last December with Dr. Ruben Niesvizky, one of the clinical directors of this center. He is incredible! He is one of those rare medical professionals who generate instant trust and respect. Then as the appointment progressed, we "clicked." He wanted me to see both a dermatologist and a neurologist. I told him I was not impressed with the dermatologist I had already seen, and he promptly had an appointment made with one at Cornell.

All the appointments had to be made in January, since our previous insurance company refused to cover any of these.

In the meantime, my friend Judith Miller had told me about this podiatrist in NYC. She and her daughter had both used this unconventional podiatrist who apparently worked miracles for both of them. Her daughter is a wonderful ballet dancer, who had trained with Rafael Grigorian; Rafael is the ballet master who attempts to teach Katie and Elizabeth. Then I found out that Rafael referred Judith to this Russian podiatrist, Dr. F. Dr. F works with mere mortals such as ourselves, but he also works extensively with dancers, ballet dancers, ice skaters, and other members of the artistic and sports communities.

So . . . I take the bus to NYC to see Dr. F. Then I see Dr. F, who looks like a cross between a gorgeous male glamour model and a lead member of some organized crime unit. I take my binder of medical history out and tell him about MGUS. He listens for about thirty seconds, takes the binder, slams it on the floor, and claims loudly "This eez boulesheet!" I am thinking to myself, how fast can I grab the binder and flee? Then he washes my feet and starts a thorough examination. He says I have frayed all five ligaments in my right foot and that the left foot is showing signs of damage. He takes X-rays in this examination room, with no shielding. I am thinking to myself, *He is mad, he is mad, mad, mad.* He measures me for orthotics, which are made based on the cast he expertly makes. Then he takes out a syringe that looks like it could be used on elephants. I told him I had a steroid shot in Binghamton that did nothing—and he asks me if the podiatrist took X-rays, and if not, how did he know where to inject the steroids? Another few "boulesheets" later, in goes the syringe (even though I thought I would see the needle point on the other side of my foot, it didn't hurt). Then he wrapped my foot. The minute the wrap went on, the pain stopped! That afternoon, I walked thirty blocks! Eventually, I walked back to my room at the very hip Hudson Hotel, showered, and slept a deep and wonderful sleep. Dr. F is truly an extraordinary podiatrist.

I woke up the next morning, got out of bed, and ended up kneeling on the floor! I had not walked any sort of distance in so long, I felt as if I had run a major marathon the day before (although we are not speaking here from any personal past experience). My muscles screamed, my body ached, and I had to laugh about the situation as I ended up in the fetal position on the floor.

I hobbled to see Dr. Niesvizky, my second visit with him. I am ten minutes late. On the ground floor, there is a gift shop. I am starving, so I stop to buy a granola bar. Standing in line, granola bar in hand, I realize Dr. Niesvizky is in line ahead of me, also with a snack bar in hand. I say hello, he asks why I am not upstairs waiting for him. I ask him why *he* isn't waiting for *me*. He says it is so busy, he didn't have time to eat. He says it is my turn to answer his question. I tell him I knew he was so busy I was buying him a granola bar!

When I see him again upstairs, I relayed the story of the extraordinary experience chez le podiatrist. We followup with the list of upcoming appointments made. When Dr. Niesvizky heard that it would be three months before I could see a neurologist back at home, he looked at me, and roared "This is boulesheet!" He picked up the phone, and before you know it, I have an appointment with a neurologist at Cornell in two weeks.

I get home and, to a much amazed family, dance a jig! Dr. F's temporary wrap is amazing!

I am going back to NYC to see the dermatologist and the neurologist next week.

*Love,*
*Olivia*

From: Olivia Chin (oliviac@yahoo.com)     Sent: 01/28/2009 7:58 AM
To: "Nick You"; "Felicia"
Cc:
Subject: "More B******t"

Dear Felicia and Nicky,

I am still smiling; I cannot wipe the silly grin from my face. It is good to
know that respected members of the medical profession in NYC have
firmly grounded funny bones and huge hearts.

I went to NYC to see various doctors. My first appointment is with Dr.
L., neurologist. She takes one of the most comprehensive histories and
Q&A sessions ever, examines me, and then asks me if I can come back
for a nerve conduction test next week. I guess my face fell because it is
such a long trip, and the hotel charges are adding up. She hops out, I hear
a discussion in the hallway, and she comes back and tells me they can
do it right away. As it turns out, her technician gave up her lunch hour
to squeeze me in. The nerve conduction test completed, Dr. L. explains
the various potential causes for the neuropathy in my foot and suggests
a seural nerve biopsy with a neurosurgeon. She asks me to ask Dr. W, the
dermatologist, about leprosy. Leprosy? How does one contract leprosy in
a small village in semi-rural upstate New York?

Then I head back to Dr. F, who rewraps my foot. Aahh! Instant relief! I
hug this guy!

My third appointment is with Dr. W, dermatologist. He looks me over,
asks me comprehensive questions about my foot and leg. He is intrigued
by the special wrap on my foot, which is a temporary orthotic. I relay
the Dr. F experience. So far, I am really impressed with every physician
at Cornell; they all take such complete pictures. After it is all done, he
gives me a prescription for a cream. And with a deadpan delivery, he says
as he leaves the room, "Leprosy? Boulesheet."

*Love,*
*Olivia*

From: Olivia Chin (oliviac@yahoo.com)   Sent: 02/11/2009 1:10 PM
To: "Nick You"
Cc:
Subject: 12 Degrees above Zero

Dear Nicky,

It is still cold.

You wanted my notes from the doctors. See the attachment.

See you next month!

*Love,*
*Olivia*

Attachment: Q&A with Dr. Niesvizky

1) Why is electrophoresis the "best" test? What is the significance of the lambda or kappa chains and their ratio?

   The normal immunoglobulin (antibody) protein structure consists of a connected pair of heavy chains (types are A, G, D, E, M) with another pair of light chains (types are kappa or lambda). In MGUS or myeloma, these immunoglobulins are not produced normally, so extra light chains can float around in the blood. In your case, you are producing more lambda chains, disconnected, which is abnormal.

2) I now have two different and conflicting results on my foot pain, one from a neurologist, one from a podiatrist. Now what?

   Both results may be right—one diagnosis does not rule out the other. There may not be a conflict of opinions. The PET-CT scan will show if there are any lesions or osteoarthritis.

3) Can you tell me about the results of the urine test from my last visit?

There is high protein in your urine, but the levels are not dangerous yet. Limit the use of ibuprofen prescribed by the podiatrist.

4) What is the projection of MGUS and the transition to myeloma for me? Is there any deterministic data?

There is no projection based on age, race, or gender. You have only one risk identified so far, the level and size of the lambda protein and the associated IgG level. The risk for MGUS progressing to myeloma is about 1 percent per year. However tests and results are pending, so let's wait to see the results of the biopsy and the PET-CT scan. After those tests are done, I would like to see you once a month for three months, and then let's see if we can reduce the frequency of your visits.

5) You said Asian females with myeloma are rare. How rare?

Out of hundreds or thousands of patients, I currently have about seven Asian females. Two of these have had high exposure to hair dye.

Attachment: Q&A with Dr. L.

The results of the nerve conduction test indicate that my nerves are demyelinating. What is the impact of this? What are the causes?

The impact of the demyelization is both motor and sensory. You only perceive the sensory impact now.

Possible causes include:
- Diabetes: I think this is unlikely since it is not bilateral
- MGUS
- CIDP: Chronic immune disorder
- Vasculitis

This is my summary of the discussion I had with Dr. L:

| Cause | Diagnosis & Method | Physician | Treatment | Owego or NYC |
|-------|-------------------|-----------|-----------|--------------|
| Diabetes | Diabetic neuropathy Method by elimination | Family physician | Medication and diet | Owego |
| MGUS | MGUS or myeloma Biopsy | Dr. B for test Dr. Niesvizky for treatment | Chemotherapy | NYC |
| CIDP | Biopsy | Dr. B for test | IV administered immunoglobulins | NYC |
| Vasculitis | Blood test | Dr. L. | Steroids | NYC |

# A DIFFICULT DIAGNOSIS: MEDICAL PERSPECTIVE

Sometimes, getting to an accurate diagnosis takes a very long time. This is especially true in relatively rare diseases, such as myeloma, with unusual presentations (foot pain) as described in Olivia's case above.

There are three cardinal findings that must be seen to make a diagnosis of multiple myeloma:

1) Greater than 10 percent plasma cells in a biopsy. The biopsy is usually of the bone marrow, but can also be from a discrete mass in the body called a plasmacytoma.
2) An M-spike in the blood or urine.
3) Organ dysfunction. Doctors are fond of acronyms since we have to memorize so much about disease and the human body. The acronym for the disease-defining organ dysfunction seen in multiple myeloma is **CRAB**: High **Calcium** level, **Renal** (kidney) insufficiency, **Anemia**, and lytic **Bone** disease.

Two out of three of the above criteria does NOT give the diagnosis of myeloma. Given that the diagnosis carries such implications in terms of deciding to give chemotherapy or proceeding with stem cell transplantation, it is important to carefully account for all three factors before telling someone that they have the disease.

The tests that your doctor needs to perform if the diagnosis of myeloma is suspected include the following:

- Thorough medical history and physical exam: to look for concerning symptoms
- Complete blood cell count: to check for anemia

- Blood electrolyte and chemistry levels: to check for abnormalities in kidney function and calcium level
- Serum protein electrophoresis (SPEP) and immunofixation (IFE), free kappa and lambda light chain levels, twenty-four-hour urine collection for Bence Jones protein, and quantitative immunoglobulin levels. (These tests are explained in more detail below.)
- Radiologic imaging of the body, either plain X-rays of the bones (skeletal survey), MRI, or PET scan, to check for the presence of lytic bone lesions. These are areas of bone that have been destroyed by multiple myeloma and have a hole-like appearance in bone.
- Bone marrow biopsy: to check for excess plasma cells and, if present in high numbers, any DNA chromosomal mutations that they can have. Certain DNA mutations in myeloma can prognostic better or worse clinical outcomes.

In a nutshell, the purpose of the SPEP, IFE, free kappa and lambda light chain levels, and twenty-four-hour urine collection are to determine the type and amount of M-protein that the myeloma plasma cells may be making. In a serum protein electrophoresis, blood serum (the stuff from blood that is left over when the red and white blood cells are removed, along with any clotting factors) is run through an agarose gel across an electrical current. This forces separation of the different protein components of plasma into several distinct visible bands, shown on the following page:

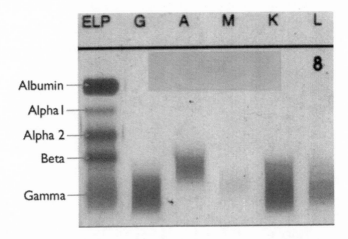

The leftmost lane of the gel called the serum protein electrophoresis. This lane is impregnated with a stain that will give all proteins a blue color nonspecifically. The dark band on top is albumin, one of the most common and abundant proteins in the bloodstream. The bands below each have names; alpha-1, alpha-2, beta, and gamma as marked in the figure.

Different blood components tend to aggregate in the different protein bands. For example, the HDL type of cholesterol runs in the band labeled alpha-2. All of the immunoglobulins run in the broad gamma band. The reason that the band is wide and fuzzy is that there are many different types of immunoglobulin proteins of different shapes and sizes, ranging from the small IgG subtype to the larger IgM subtype, and each runs slightly different on the gel.

The same serum sample is run through the other lanes labeled G, A, M, K, and L shown above. These lanes constitute the immunofixation. Each of these lanes is impregnated with a specific stain that will mark only one type of protein specifically. In the "G" lane, it is the immunoglobulin type G antibody, in the "A" lane, it is the immunoglobulin type A, etc. For K and L, the stains will mark the kappa and lambda light chains respectively. In the normal human sample above, we see that the darkest bands are seen in the G and K lanes—this is because we tend to have more immunoglobulin type G and kappa light chains as compared to the other types. Still, the bands in each lane are wide and fuzzy, meaning that even within the specific subtypes of antibody, there is a variation in shape and size, because different molecules are produced by a variety of different plasma cells normally.

In the serum protein electrophoresis/immunofixation from a person with a monoclonal paraprotein (see below), the gamma band is narrowed and sharp. There is now one predominant kind of immunoglobulin (called the monoclonal immunoglobulin) that runs at one precise spot on the gel, giving rise to the famous M-spike. By looking at the immunofixation lanes, we can easily see a prominent sharp band in the M and L lanes. This signifies that in this case, the M-protein produced is the IgM-lambda subtype. This M-spike can be measured and followed throughout the clinical course of an individual and roughly reflects the amount of malignant plasma cells in the body. A rapidly rising M-protein connotes aggressive growing myeloma, while falling or disappearing M-protein can signify a good response to treatment.

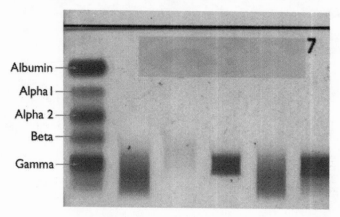

The most common presenting symptoms of multiple myeloma are back pain and fatigue. The back pain is usually due to a compression fracture of one of the vertebral bodies (the bones that make up the bulk of your spine). The fatigue may come from either anemia or kidney problems. As more and more plasma cells take up space in the bone marrow, there is less room for normal blood elements to live and function; this leads to the anemia. As those plasma cells secrete more immunoglobulin (the M-protein) into the blood, these proteins become too much for the kidney to handle, leading to a situation like hair getting clogged in a drain. It is important to avoid any medications that may hamper kidney function in myeloma. These include non-steroidal inflammatory drugs (NSAIDs), such as ibuprofen and naproxen.

Rarely, myeloma may present with recurrent infections like pneumonias or skin abscesses due to excess abnormal immunoglobulin squeezing out the normal protective ones that should be a part of a healthy immune system. Persons with myeloma may also first notice either a loss of sensation, tingling, or uncomfortable feeling in the legs or hands due to neuropathy.

When Olivia first came to her doctors for help, the M-protein was present, but she did not have the level of plasma cells necessary nor did she have any of the CRAB features that would have easily led to the diagnosis of myeloma. Given the availability of the information at the time, she was given the correct diagnosis of MGUS. It is to her credit (and her doctors) that this was not the end of the story and a continuing investigation was made into alternative diagnoses that could be leading to her foot pain and increasing fatigue at home.

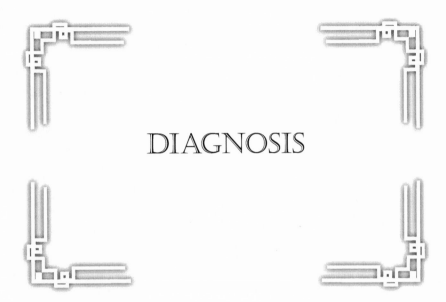

# DIAGNOSIS

From: Olivia Chin (oliviac@yahoo.com)   Sent: 02/14/2009 11:58 PM
To: "Nick You"; "Felicia"
Cc:
Subject: Biopsy

Dear Felicia and Nicky,

I am hobbling around and using a scooter, having had the biopsy on the right ankle. Dr. B, the neurosurgeon, took out a section of nerve and muscle. It hurts! It also takes eight to ten days to get the results, so I am patiently waiting.

The night before the biopsy, Wai and I checked into an elegant boutique hotel. Thanks to the recession, we are able to book hotels for less. Wai is happy to watch the large-screen TV. I decide to go to the Disney store to trade Disney collectible pins and skip dinner, Wai reluctantly comes along. So we go, trade pins, and come back to the hotel, chilled to the bone. It was extremely cold, a penetrating, damp cold. I hobble to take a steamy shower and then snuggle in the foam memory bed, covered with an eiderdown. The heat is on high, and I am staring out the almost floor-to-ceiling window. The view of the Manhattan skyline is breathtaking. I ask Wai how he is doing, as my eyes get heavy. He says he is still cold, he is hungry, the bed is hard, the TV is at a bad angle, and he is miserable. He asks me how I am feeling. I tell him "This is bliss." We are obviously made for each other!

The morning of the biopsy, my blood sugar was so high that the anesthesiologists refused me. I do not understand—I had been fasting since three p.m. the day before. How could my glucose be that high? So we did it, using just a local. I have had more pleasant experiences.

Do you know the positive outcome of not going under? You can eat right after.

Just lucky I guess.

Love,
Olivia

From: Olivia Chin (oliviac@yahoo.com)   Sent: 02/24/2009 8:42 PM
To: Friendlist
Cc:
Subject: Happy New Year!

Dear Friends,

Since the last e-mail, I had the PET-CT scan, a nerve conduction test, a biopsy, and three or four more trips to NYC. They have now eliminated syphilis and leprosy at this time. Whew! I have weird rashes from head to foot, numb spots, numb toes, blisters, and pain. Pain is an amazing thing—it can zap you of energy, it can put a damper of even the happiest moments, and it mostly just makes me want to bite the person closest to me. I now have a scooter to zip around the house on bad days. Come on over! I might chase you, run you over, and then bite. I would love to have company, really.

*Mi casa es su casa. Crunch.*

I have good news and bad news. Last Friday I called Wai from NYC and told him that the good news is that I had just got a diagnosis as the result of the sural nerve and muscle biopsy. The bad news is that I have AL amyloidosis, and the treatment is chemo and stem cell replacement therapy (SCRT). By Sunday, I viewed it differently. The bad news is I have AL amyloidosis, and its mortality rate is fairly high. The good news is that there is a treatment plan, and its mortality rate is low. I do not know yet what the success rate is, but the options are so limited it doesn't matter. Three weeks ago, I had a biopsy of the seural nerve and muscle tissue. The diagnosis of the nerve biopsy shows amyloid due to immunoglobulin deposition around the blood vessels of peripheral nerves. The deep muscle results show mild neurogenic atrophy. In English, this means that those excess proteins that showed up previously in the blood and urine are unprocessed, and they are infiltrating tissues they should not, causing damage and inflammation. I was told that amyloidosis is rare and that there are many different types. People with amyloid get sick due to accumulation of the amyloid protein in various places in their bodies, such as the skin, nerves, and organs. They told me that based on the evidence accumulated thus far, my type of amyloid is called AL; it is the light chain part of the immunoglobulin molecule that is building up and causing damage in my nerves.

*I always hated organic chem.*

There is no cure, but there is treatment. Treatment focuses on lessening symptoms and production of amyloid. The treatment, if I am eligible, will be chemo and SCRT. I don't think I have significant damage yet to any organs, so we'll see. The SCRT will be autologous, which means they collect my stem cells, filter them, kill my stem cells (and immune system), and then put them back in and wait for them to come back around and rebuild my immune. This is sort of like reloading the operating system on a PC. Isn't it amazing that we have a built-in reboot kit in our bodies? I go back to NYC again next Friday to get more information. For those of you more curious, try www.amyloidosis.org. There is also information on the Mayo Clinic, Cleveland Clinic, and Sloan Kettering websites.

*I'd rather go on a cruise.*

So, this means lots more trips to NYC. Lots more restaurants to try. Lots more rich men I get to meet (too bad they are all doctors). I believe wine, chocolate, and curry are still very important! I will let you all know what comes up next—and an approximate timetable of events. I am so grateful to Dr. Ruben Niesvizky, Clinical Director of the MM group at Cornell medical. When the local hematologist in Broome Oncology said the course of action was to monitor the MGUS two to three times a year, Dr. Niesvizky kept plugging along. While I think the local doctors are fine, Dr. Niesvizky is in a class by himself. As far as I am concerned, he is a god amongst men. His staff is amazing too. He has introduced me to one of his colleagues, Dr. Tomer Mark. These two men are going to save my life or at least prolong it.

*I hope neither of them had to retake organic chem like somebody we know.*

Otherwise, we're okay. The girls are holding up well, taking on additional responsibilities around the house, and getting better grades than I ever did. Between them, they handle the dog, laundry, dishes, and restocking the toilet paper supply. Katie has learned to make grilled cheese (goat cheese and gluten-free bread). Due to her food intolerances (wheat, dairy, eggs), I spent Sunday cooking and putting frozen lunches and dinners away.

*Eat. Drink. Man. Woman.*

My mother now knows. I have this to say—every decision, every appointment, every step of the way seems to have been guided. Getting Niesvizky as my doctor. The local neurologist was not available for months, so Dr. Niesvizky had me see one in NYC (Dr. L.). She was instrumental in the first step toward diagnosis. When she reversed her decision on the biopsy, I disagreed with her whether to proceed with it. My GP (Dr. R) came up with the one piece of data that didn't "jive", which convinced her to proceed with the biopsy. I disagreed with the neurosurgeon which foot to use for the biopsy and had it done under local when the anesthesiologists refused to put me under. Even the switch in insurance companies and when appointments around that change were scheduled was fortuitous.

*Luck and pluck. The divine and wine.*

If you want to help, send good vibes my way! I pray often for a friend who is also undergoing chemo and SCRT, and I send positive thoughts her way. It may sound hokey, but will you all do it for me? Also, I may turn to all of you for help at one point or another as I have already when going to NY. I am grateful to and for all of you, my circle of friends. You are my adopted family.

*Send money!*

Love,
Olivia

From: Olivia Chin (oliviac@yahoo.com)     Sent: 02/24/2008 9:57 PM
To: "Nick You"
Cc:
Subject: Told Mom. My turn to rant and rave.

Dear Nicky,

I finally told Mom. It was really hard. I am so mad. I told her gently that I have bone marrow cancer—it was easier than amyloidosis. She started ranting and raving about how she should never have lived to be so old. I had no idea what she was talking about, so I kept quiet and listened. Then it comes out: "I should never have lived to be so old. Now I have to see my child die before me!"

*I can arrange for that not to happen. You could die sooner than expected.*

I told her I had no immediate plans to die. But she outsmarted me. She changed her tactics. She started saying how she had me when she was too old, that this is all her fault, and this is why I have cancer. She feels so guilty. She never should have had me so late in her life.

*I can arrange for the guilt to stop rather instantly.*

Mom is ninety, she is so fit and active, and she is also not going to change. So I listen, and then I leave, go home, and cry. I wanted to be comforted. I wanted a cup of hot tea. I wanted Mom to tell me she loves me and that everything will be all right. Instead, I got a self-centered, raving woman, and I could not wait to go. I wanted to scream: "THIS IS NOT ABOUT YOU!" I wanted to be the self-centered raving woman!

So, I have come up with the top ten things NOT to say to someone who has cancer:

1.  How are you feeling? *While this greeting is fine for when undergoing intensive treatment, it takes a toll over an extended period of time. This is a not a typical address. Last I knew, I was still Olivia Chin, not Cancer Chin. Whatever happened to "Hi! What are you up to?" or "What are you doing?" or "What's new with you?" It would be lovely*

*to have a conversation that does not always come back to my health status like a boomerang.*

2. When do you see the doctor next? When do you get test results back? *There is a reason for HIPPA. It is my choice when and whether I share this with you. Also, waiting for test results is nerve-wracking. If I didn't get the results back yet, I may not want to think about it or be reminded of it. And if I did, perhaps I am just not ready yet to share them. Either way, you lose. This is as bad as, "Are you pregnant?"*

3. Do you know why you have this? How did you get this? *If I did something to get cancer, I still do not deserve cancer. There is no answer to this question for me. I do not fit the typical profiles. So, the next time someone asks me that question, I plan to answer with, "Yes, it's because I am really an African American male cross-dresser, and I was exposed to Agent Orange when I was twelve years old and a soldier in Vietnam!" Geesh! And if I did do something stupid that brought this on, why would I want to be reminded of it and share it with you?*

4. I thought something like cancer was up, you look sooo tired. *The only person I know who made tired look sooo good was Madeline Kahn, when she crooned as Lili von Shtupp "I'm so tired, of being admired! I'm so tired, of being desired." If you thought something was up, you must be a medical phenomenon, since the twenty or so physicians I have seen over the last eighteen months were unable to figure it out ... Besides, I thought I was looking pretty good. Since when does anyone want to hear they look tired anyway? ("Are you pregnant?")*

5. Phone message: "OMG I am so sorry, I just heard. OMG, I feel terrible, I don't know what to say, I don't know what to do. I couldn't sleep last night when I heard. OMG. Can I walk the dog for you? I'll come and scrub your toilets if you need me to. OMG. I feel so bad." *This is an actual phone message someone left me! This is not about **you**. I am so sorry **you** feel so bad, and **you** couldn't sleep. I hope it wears off. I did not mean for my cancer to cause you such anguish. BTW, please keep your neurosis to yourself. My dog*

*is doing fine; I have a husband and two kids who walk him. AND MY TOILETS ARE CLEAN, THANK YOU!*

6. Phone message: "Call me back; I want to know your status. People are asking me about you, and I need to know what to tell them. I really need to know." *This is another real message that was left on my voice mail. There are people who are information junkies. And there are people who are busybodies who want to tell everyone stuff about me. My close friends and family know. I have picked a friend to be a spokesperson for me. You are not the chosen one.*

7. So are you cured? *I just recently learned that many cancers have no cure. Once a cancer, always a cancer. However, there are various stages of cancer. One could be in remission or not. A few lucky ones experience complete remission. Dr. Mark made a remarkable comparison between cancer and other diseases recently that I found enlightening. He said we could think of cancer as a more formidable cousin of diabetes or hypertension. Do we ask a diabetic if he is cured? Do we ask a person with high blood pressure if her treatment is working? I realize some cancers have poor survival statistics—but, please, this question just hurts.*

8. You should try mangosteen juice . . . Have you looked into this clinical trial? *Do I look like a freaking idiot? I have looked into everything available on the Internet. Judging from the stack of my bedside books, it would appear I am going to medical school. I have charted my markers. I have a database of my test results. I have read medical papers from over the last decade (most of which I do not understand). I am seeking the best medical help I can. Please don't tell me that I can cure this by wrapping my left arm around my head while sucking wild blueberries soaked in green tea extract while chanting "The rain in Spain stays mainly on the plain."*

9. Do you know Mike S? I think he has the same thing as you. He's home now in hospice care. I hear he is in terrible pain. And did you know Sylvia C? She died last year, but I think she had the same cancer. *Need I say anything more?*

10. Silence. *The most hurtful of all are those who won't or can't deal with me anymore.*

Sniff. Pass the tissues please.

I feel much better now!

*Love,*
*Olivia*

From: Olivia Chin (oliviac@yahoo.com)    Sent: 02/26/2009 9:28 AM
To: "Nick You"; "Felicia"
Cc:
Subject: Love and marriage

Dear Felicia and Nicky,

I am so mad! Can you believe Wai? He made an appointment to see our lawyer, and he asked me how I wanted to be buried. I told him that after twenty-six and a half years of marriage, I think it odd that I know exactly how he wants to be buried, but he forgot what I wanted! I also told him it would be nice if he would focus on my treatment and recovery rather than my demise. Oh, well . . .

I am thinking I could arrange his burial in the immediate future . . . but then, shucks, he has to live. I need the medical benefits! Okay, scratch that thought!

So I reminded him that I wanted to be cremated and that two years after my death, he should go on a singles cruise and throw the ashes overboard. He asked me how he should do that with two young kids in tow. I think that is his problem.

So, I thought the ancient Egyptians had a good thing—and told Wai I could be buried in a beautiful tomb, along with him next to me. We could entomb some of my cookie jars along with us. It would kill two birds with one stone (bad pun), and he wouldn't have to worry about his own burial.

He said he didn't intend to build me a tomb.

So, then I told him perhaps the Hindu warriors had it right. I could be burnt, and he could be burnt right next to me on the pyre. I grinned at him and said "Burn with me baby! Burn."

At that point, he walked out of the room.

You know, marriage just isn't what it used to be.

Love,
Olivia

# DIAGNOSIS:
# MEDICAL PERSPECTIVE

At the end of a long process of medical testing and waiting, Olivia had been diagnosed with a rare disease called AL amyloidosis. Amyloidosis is an umbrella term for a kind of illness that results from the deposition of a protein in various places in the body, such as the heart, lungs, brain, kidneys, or skin. Any disease in which an abnormally folded protein deposits in an organ and causes health problems can be called a type of amyloidosis. Amyloid syndromes are defined by the type of protein that accumulates and there are many different kinds. A few of the more common types are listed in the table below:

| Amyloid Disease | Misfolded Protein | Organ Affected |
|---|---|---|
| Familial Amyloid | Mutated Transthyretin protein— Transthyretin is a protein that is normally made in the liver; it functions as a chaperone of thyroid hormone, among other things | Heart, Nerves |
| Senile Amyloid | Transthyretin—unmutated type | Heart |
| Dialysis-Associated Amyloid | Beta-2 Microglobulin—this is a protein that is normally involved in the immune system self-recognition process and is normally excreted by the kidney | Joints |
| Inflammation-associated | Serum AA protein—increases in inflammation; sustained prolonged elevations seen with chronic infections (e.g. hepatitis) and rheumatologic disease (e.g. rheumatoid arthritis) | Kidneys |

| AL (primary) Amyloid | Immunoglobulin light chain | Heart, kidneys, lungs, skin, nerves |
|---|---|---|
| Alzheimer's disease | Beta Amyloid Protein | Brain |

If not inherently obvious, such as in the case of Alzheimer disease, the diagnosis of amyloidosis can be difficult to make. The diagnostic process takes several steps. First, amyloid deposition in an organ/tissue must be demonstrated with a biopsy; second, the type of amyloid must be determined; third, a review of affected organs must take place. A biopsy of a target organ is most telling, however, it is often inconvenient or impractical to biopsy a heart, kidney, or nerve. What is usually done is biopsy of a surrogate site where amyloid can accumulate. Most often this is the abdominal fat pad, rectum, or gums. The biopsy is stained with a dye called Congo red. Amyloid stained with Congo red will glow when looked at through polarized light in an effect called apple-green birefringence.

The type of amyloid is sometimes difficult to determine. If available, mass spectrometry or electron gold microscopy demonstrating small fibrils of protein infiltrating the body tissue can be helpful. Often, the clinical scenario is what informs the most. In Olivia's case, her blood work showed an elevation of the lambda free light chain (see prior section on myeloma) and a bone marrow biopsy that showed a small clonal population of plasma cells that also expressed a predominance of lambda light chain protein. Her nerve biopsy also stained positively for the accumulation and deposition of lambda light chain. Given this data, it was evident that she had AL (also called primary) amyloidosis. Lambda light chain has a particular propensity to form amyloid (lambda outnumbers kappa AL amyloid by about 4 to 1). AL amyloid should always be suspected when a patient is diagnosed with a new lambda light chain type myeloma, as they can coexist approximately 10 percent of the time. Without evidence for a culprit light chain, AA (inflammatory type) and inherited amyloidoses become possibilities. A long history of infection or autoimmune illness, such as rheumatoid arthritis, can point towards AA. A family history of cardiac disease and an African

American background can hint at the possibility of the inherited type of amyloidosis.

AL amyloidosis can have a variable clinical course of illness, depending on the severity of deposition and involved organs. For instance, one person may have heart involvement only, another kidney and nerve involvement, another with lung and skin involvement, etc. While not exactly known yet, scientists postulate that the particular protein sequence of the responsible lambda light chain determines where it will be deposited (described in a term called *tropism*). When first diagnosed, the physician should search conduct diagnostic testing to look for which organs may be affected with studies such as breathing studies, echocardiography, and blood work amongst other tests.

In Olivia's case, she had nerve involvement. Extensive medical workup was performed, including looking at heart function and lung function, and fortunately she escaped significant amyloid deposition in other parts of her body for the most part. Extent of organ, especially heart, involvement is the most telling prognostic factor for persons with AL amyloidosis. For instance, people with a significant cardiac burden can have nearly half the life expectancy and may not be eligible for riskier interventions, such as stem cell transplantation (discussed in more detail in an upcoming section).

There can be significant confusion in separating a diagnosis of AL amyloidosis from multiple myeloma. Recall the definition of myeloma given in the previous section: 1) plasma cells accumulation; 2) M-protein in the blood or urine; 3) CRAB features. Persons with AL amyloidosis have the M-protein component and often a small level of plasmacytosis in the bone marrow, but no CRAB features. One way to think of AL amyloid is as a form of myeloma with a low tumor cell burden. Normally, the low numbers of tumor cells cause no harm in a person other than production of the M-protein and the disease state would be classified as an MGUS. With time, the plasma cell population grows and CRAB end-organ dysfunction may arise, leading to an evolving myeloma. In AL amyloid, *the M-protein itself is the problem,* not the plasma cells. Significant health problems develop before myeloma in its proper sense can seen. Between 5-15 percent of patients with multiple myeloma have AL amyloid as well.

The overlap between AL amyloidosis and multiple myeloma supports the idea that these two diseases may be on the same spectrum.

There are challenges that the physician faces in delivering the news of an AL amyloidosis diagnosis to a patient. One is that being a rare disease, most doctors have only read about it in textbooks way back in medical school, where it was often described as a vague fatal disease with bleak prospects for treatment. Lack of knowledge may lead to inability to fully communicate what amyloidosis is and what it means to the patient. This leads to more questions than answers. The second challenge also lies in terms of general ignorance on the subject. If most doctors have only passing knowledge that the disease exists, you can only imagine that the majority of the public at large has absolutely no idea what AL amyloidosis is. This led to some stress for Olivia. While she was surrounded by caring friends and family, their attempts to help often led to her having to explain amyloid, her treatment options, and her outlook to them. This is tough to do when your major resource is the Internet, where it seems that it is the people with bad experiences that feel most motivated to communicate what AL amyloid is to the world. With the right circumstances and treatment, AL amyloid is highly treatable with a reasonably good long-term outcome and life expectancy. A caring, knowledgeable doctor and the right support group of patients/families affected by amyloidosis can be crucial at the outset of coming to terms with a new diagnosis.

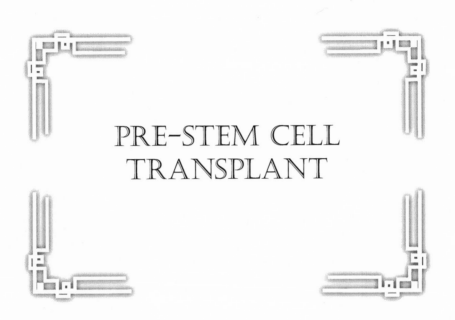

# PRE-STEM CELL
# TRANSPLANT

From: Olivia Chin (oliviac@yahoo.com)     Sent: 03/11/09 10:49 PM
To: Friendlist
Cc:
Subject: No Free Margaritas

Dear Friends,

It looks like a stem cell transplant may be in my future. I have done some reading, and we have had some initial discussions with Dr. Mark at Weill-Cornell. Dr. Mark takes over from Dr. Niesvizky once the decision is made to proceed with a stem cell transplant. From what I can gather, this is an all-inclusive weight loss program, except there are rampant rumors about the food being really, really lousy, and even worse, there are no free, all-you-can-drink margaritas.

Dr. Niesvizky suggested that I go for a second opinion to a specialist in Boston. Another trip, another hotel, another doctor. Sigh. I wasn't able to get an appointment in Boston right away. Deep sigh.

There are times when it is hard. I surprised myself when I cried myself to sleep one night. It might have been right after we went to the lawyer and updated our wills, our health care proxies, our "do not resuscitate" orders, and our power of attorney forms. These updates were long overdue. Given the circumstances, it was difficult.

I want to see Katie and Elizabeth grow up. I want to help them find their niche. I want to meet the people who are going to give them long-lasting happiness. I want to see my grandchildren—in due time. I want to spend a lot more time showing Wai how much I care about him. Five simple wishes.

If you stop to think about it, we all have just a handful of simple wishes.

*Love,*
*Olivia*

From: Olivia Chin (oliviac@yahoo.com)      Sent: 03/17/09 1:10 PM
To: Friendlist
Cc:
Subject: Margaritaville

Dear Friends,

The stem cell transplant will probably start in six weeks or so, which means I will be in NYC for several days before for preparation, and then down there for a three week hospital stay. After being discharged, I am hoping to stay in NYC for awhile until my immune system builds up enough to come home. The doctors are worried about the two-hundred-year-old house, the dog, and the kids still being in school. So I may be in NYC for two to three months. We are looking into a studio apartment in Manhattan, thanks to Helene, my best girlfriend from college.

I can honestly say I am scared! I cut my hair really short in anticipation of hair loss, and I look a lot like my brother right now. I am also losing weight slowly—not sure why. I am on some high fallutin' pain killers, so it is a little easier to get through the day. I am cooking large batches of food so the family can continue to eat well while I am away (what a Chinese thing to do!). I have everything organized and set up for the upcoming dance competitions for Katie and Elizabeth. I am frantically getting paperwork for insurance submittals squared away. Mostly, I am tired and sleep a lot. Another thing—the docs said to eat whatever I want now because later everything will need to be overcooked and pasteurized. I have eaten more raw shellfish and sushi in the last three weeks than I have in my entire life! Geoduck may soon be an endangered species!

Yum!

Love,
Olivia

From: Olivia Chin (oliviac@yahoo.com)     Sent: 03/18/2009 9:28 AM
To: "Nick You"
Cc:
Subject: Help

Dear Nicky,

I've been thinking. Besides Wai, the girls, and mom, you are really my only family. I know we were close growing up, but the last thirty years living on different continents has resulted in my kids trying to figure out where you fit in. We get to see you about once a year. Wai and I have continued the tradition in our children to have them address close adult friends as aunt and uncle. They are confused as to who are "friend" uncles and who is their real uncle.

Since I will be in NYC for much of the summer, and Wai does intend to continue working in order to support me in the manner to which I am accustomed to living, we have a slight problem of childcare coverage this summer.

What are your plans? Can you help at all? I have of course another reason for asking you. While I realize my children will never be the same after spending any sort of extended time with you, I would like them to get to know you, to play with you, to hear stories about me that only you can share with them.

Our lives have been such that I have never really asked you for anything until now. Please help me?

*Love,*
*Olivia*

From: Nick You　　　　　　　　　　Sent: 03/21/2009 8:12 AM
To: "Olivia Chin"
Cc:
Subject: RE: Help

Olivia,

I had no specific plans this summer. Tell me when you need me and for
how long and where? In Owego I imagine with the kids.

Just so that you know, I have separated from W★★★y. So if I come, I
will be coming with my current partner, who is older than me and is
Italian.

Do you want me to do any inquiries in China? They are most probably
the most advanced in stem cell practices.

All my strength,
Nicky

From: Olivia Chin (oliviac@yahoo.com)    Sent: 03/23/2009 7:48 AM
To: "Nick You"
Cc:
Subject: RE: Help

Dear Nicky,

Okay ... First of all, *partner* in the US means you have a gay male partner.
So please clarify. (Is he cute? Ha ha).

Two—please, please tell me you are not in another rebound relationship!
(Although you know what I thought about W★★★y). So tell him or her:
I lova pasta! I lova pizza! I lova artichokas!)

Three—I do not know what help I will need yet. I may have to stay in
NYC for up to one hundred days after discharge. Wai will stay with me
for two weeks, and then Louise for one or two weeks. I don't know if I
will have the strength yet to be able to take care of myself after three to
four weeks. So I may need you to stay in Owego and help with the kids,
who currently may be shuttled to Binghamton, the Chesapeake area, and
or even Claire's in Aigle for the summer ... or I may need you in the
NYC studio, helping me get fed, to the doctors (two times per week,
etc). If you can work out of NYC, I may only need help with groceries,
cooking, and doctor trips. (I was told I would be very, very weak). You
should know the studio is going to be kept very clean—hepa-filtered air,
AC, etc. The diet is also very strict—neutropenic. Everything pasteurized
or very washed and then overcooked. Nothing from delis, no buffets, no
fast food. Bottled spring water or boiled water only. There is a huge list
of forbidden foods. They are worried mostly about molds, mildews, and
fungi because they can medicate the heck out of anything else. So I think
that also means no baked Brie or Gorgonzola in puff pastry.

Four—please do not get married anytime soon. I do not break promises,
and right now, I cannot travel far. Remember when you got married
to W★★★y, and you asked me to come to your wedding in Southern
France with a week's notice? Well, I was in the midst of a major review
on the radar project, and I told you I was sorry I could not make it to
wedding Number Three. But I promised you I would make it to wedding

Number Four. So hold off this time until I can travel again! (I love being your younger pesky sister).

I plan to stay in the studio for three to five months. It is a nice sunny studio with a little kitchen and regular-sized bath on Fortieth Street, between Second and Third Avenues. It is really near the UN. You could walk to work.

China—I think I am too close to the procedure at this point to consider another option in terms of stem cell protocol or procedure. I am seeing another amyloidosis specialist, Dr. Comenzo, in Boston soon. He was at Sloan Kettering and moved to Tufts Medical last year. Right now, Weill-Cornell Medical is where I am going, and they are pretty up there in the multiple myeloma world. Amyloidosis is similar to MM. The only other places in the states would be the Mayo Clinic (who wants to go to Minnesota?) or Sloan Kettering. Being on the bleeding edge here also means being possibly part of a clinical trial. I decided that given my age and relative health, I do not wish to take the chance of being the group on the placebo, so China or some other place may be an option when this comes back and there are fewer options. I understand France is pretty advanced. Well, I speak the language! (Garçon! Le gâteau au chocolat noir avec le coulis au framboise s'il vous plait!) Also, this field is booming, so perhaps when it comes back, progress will have been made.

Otherwise, we're fine, a little shocked still. In all seriousness, I hope you are happy with the Italiano or Italiana. I am sending you a little something I wrote many years ago. Enjoy your parmesan. I'll settle for my beloved cottage cheese.

Love,
Olivia

# Men Are Like Cheese

*I like to compare men to cheese. I love cheese, especially cottage cheese, but I digress.*

*I remember a man who was much older than me. He was like a fine-aged Parmesan cheese, Italian, salty, sweet, and sexy, with incredible flavor and flair. It took time for the flavors to develop, but oh what flavors! Good with fine wines, he knew what to say, how to dress, where to go—a wonderful learning experience, but who wants a lifetime of education?*

*Then there was the man who I think of as my tete de moine, a pungent carrot top, stinky and odd-looking, but when you looked under the skin, what a creamy, delicious cheese! If you are lucky to have this cheese in your house, everything will reek—your entire house will smell, your clothes will smell, your hair will smell, even your skin will smell. It melts in your mouth in a rich, smooth, wonderful explosion of gooey flavor. But once a year is enough.*

*There is the type of earthy and sensual man, the spiritual kind who wears socks with sandals after summer, who usually sports a scratchy beard and an even scratchier Shetland wool sweater, and who skis and plays squash. I think of these as goat cheeses, with slightly musky undertones. There are a variety of these, some sprinkled with peppercorns or herbs, some anointed in oil. Dressing up to these means putting on a layer of straw or hay. These are good for a fling, wonderful when you have a craving for multi-grain bread smeared with a crumbly goat cheese, great for picnics in the fall outdoors, or on a blanket surrounded by trees.*

*There are the Bries and Camemberts that always look appropriate at a party served on a tray with crackers. These men I also think of as peacock males. They are rich, they look good, and they work hard at looking good and pleasing all of the women all of the time. They are not particularly interesting, but they are nice to have around. They are always preening themselves, and they are always served with crackers. Unfortunately, the woman is the cracker. Sooner or later, it gets boring.*

*There are the one-night-stand cheeses, the ones with jalapeno flakes, the Spanish hard cheeses laced with peppercorns, the soft French ones with a garlic bite, the Swiss spring milk tomes, plain-looking but rich, and the smoky Swede, unexpectedly sweet.*

*My husband is . . . cottage cheese. I could eat cottage cheese every day for the rest of my life. I can have it with fruit to zing it up. I often will eat it out of the plastic tub. It doesn't stink, I never find bits of hay in it, I don't have to be in a special mood to eat it, and it is never, ever served with crackers. I love cottage cheese. When I get old, I will still want my cottage cheese.*

From: Nick You  Sent: 03/26/2009 9:18 AM
To: "Olivia Chin"
Cc:
Subject: RE: Help

Dear Olivia,

*Italiana,* of course!

Just tell me when and where I can be of most use. I could also take care of the kids in Switzerland or in Kenya. Do you think they would be ready for a safari?

Nicky

From: Olivia Chin (oliviac@yahoo.com)    Sent: 03/27/2009 9:42 PM
To: "Nick You"
Cc:
Subject: RE: Help

Dear Nicky,

Italiana? May I recommend you to use terms like "my Italian girlfriend" or "my bella" or even "my bitch"—but *NOT* partner.

No safari. Sorry. I want to see my kids sometime. I can just see the look on Dr. Mark's face when I ask him when I can eat sushi again, and in what year I can see my kids again given they just came back from a Masai village with malaria and white spots on the undersides of their feet.

On our last trip to NYC, we brought the kids. They were all set to go to the Museum of Natural History until I let slip that I also wanted to go to Nintendo World. We spent over four hours there the first day. I refused to go with them when they took off again the next day to continue their hours of play.

We are now the proud owners of a Wii. Actually, it's on order and coming. Wai figured in the weeks to come, it would be entertainment for the girls. Methinks Wai might play the Wii a wee bit too.

*Love,*
*Olivia*

From: Larry Moss                                    Sent: 03/31/2009 1:12 PM
To: airigamiannounce@airigami.com
Cc:
Subject: Elastic Park and Balloon Manor

It's been awhile since I've sent an update on Airigami out to this list. As always, if you want to be removed from this list, just let me know.

Quite a bit has happened since the last update in the last few months with Airigami (http://www.airigami.com/) and Balloon Manor (http://www.balloonmanor.com/). Websites have both been redesigned from the ground up. It's a lot easier to see the latest photos, including one of a dress I made for Fashion Week in NYC. I've also started a new blog on Airigami.com, so you can read stories about projects and even get notified of new blog entries and learn about the latest Airigami projects (including one that I'll talk about in just a moment that makes Balloon Manor look small) via Twitter (http://twitter.com/airigami).

So what could I have going that's larger than Balloon Manor? A project that one could say has been in development for over sixty-five million years. Elastic Park, a reproduction of Jurassic Park, is coming soon. If you're a Facebook user, you can become a fan of Elastic Park by visiting http://www.facebook.com/pages/New-York-NY/Elastic-Park/55706635818

Here's the story I posted about it on my blog:
"Any other time, we'd let you see the space. But today there are elephants in the way." That's not the sort of thing you typically hear when booking an event. Or at least I don't. But maybe people that play places like Madison Square Garden are used to that. After hearing it, my mind raced back and forth a bit between a deep frustration that I wasn't able to see the space I'd be working in right at that moment and the thought, "Who cares? I'm getting to do an installation in Madison Square Garden."

Yeah, that's right. The largest Airigami installation to date will appear this coming year in the Expo Center at MSG. Elastic Park, a recreation of Michael Crichton's Jurassic Park, will be built, entirely out of balloons. Mark Verge, a fantastic artist that I've been working with for years on Balloon Manor (and other projects) has been working for some time on dinosaurs. We've been talking for awhile about creating them at the scale and in the environment they should be. Finally, with the help of NBC Universal, we're going to do it right. One hundred thousand balloons, a 36,000-square-foot venue, and forty artists will honor the late Michael Crichton.

The largest Airigami projects have always benefited health-related charities. This one is no different. Mr. Crichton passed away from cancer just recently. Many Airigami crew members have experienced cancer in their families. We've teamed up with the American Cancer Society to present the latest of our projects, and we're looking forward to raising a lot of money for an organization that does so much good. All money from ticket sales will go directly to the American Cancer Society's Hope Lodge.

Larry Moss, http://www.airigami.com
PO Box 23523, Rochester, NY 14692, (585) 359-8695
Airigami: The fine art of folding air

From: Olivia Chin (oliviac@yahoo.com)　Sent: 04/02/2009 10:42 AM
To: "Larry Moss"
Cc:
Subject: RE: Elastic Park and Balloon Manor

Larry,

I may actually be using Hope Lodge in May or June!

I was diagnosed with AL amyloidosis in March. I am starting my stem cell collection next week, and hope to go through the stem cell transplant at Weill-Cornell Medical, which is affiliated with New York Presbyterian Hospital in NYC in early May. Hope Lodge is the facility mentioned to us by the hospital social worker and transplant coordinator that we may want to use upon discharge. I have been working with the Multiple Myeloma Clinic at Cornell since December, and they are an amazing group of people.

Let me know if I can help in any way. I did my undergrad in NYC at NYU back in the age of the dinosaurs (ha ha) and am still familiar with the city and restaurants. Although I will be immune-compromised for many months, I would like to think I can help with another Airigami project.

Can I suggest something for you to consider? Is there a time slot first thing one morning for perhaps one hour, when the air has cleared out overnight, when you could open this exhibit to only those people who are undergoing chemo or stem cell transplants, or any who have immune issues (HIV, etc)? It would be incredible publicity, too. This could involve kids and adults, and considering where this is held, you could possibly attract people from the tri-state area. If the American Cancer Society or some TV show spotlights this, I'll bet you would have an interesting turnout.

I want to be first in line with a paid ticket!

Love,
Olivia

From: Larry Moss                                    Sent: 04/03/2009 11:15 AM
To: "Olivia Chin"
Cc:
Subject: Re: Elastic Park and Balloon Manor

Olivia,

We talked a lot in October about your health. I had hoped things were better by now. It sounds like things have just progressed at this point. I'm sorry you need to use Hope Lodge, but I'm really glad it's there for you. It's a great place, and the people I've met there are fantastic.

When things are really underway, I'm putting the whole crew in a hotel within a few blocks of MSG. You know what the build can be like. And on this build, we only have four days, so it will be pretty insane. Come join us if you can!

I love the idea of having a special time for people at Hope Lodge or others through ACS that can't go when the large crowds are there. I expect that would be a real problem to arrange once we open, but I'd love to do that as a preview, maybe during the last build day. I'd also love to have you walk that group through as someone who has been on one of my build crews. We'll be scrambling to finish, so we won't be able to stop and talk much, but if I gave you the script and even audio recordings, they'll get something really cool out of it, and they'd be performing a test run before we open. Anyway, they will be able to see the final stages of the build.

Let me know how you are doing.

Larry Moss, http://www.airigami.com
PO Box 23523, Rochester, NY 14692, (585) 359-8695
Airigami: The fine art of folding air

From: Olivia Chin (oliviac@yahoo.com)   Sent: 04/06/2009 11:12 AM
To: "Larry Moss"
Cc:
Subject: RE: Elastic Park and Balloon Manor

Larry,

It would be an honor to lead this group through Elastic Park.

I'm actually doing pretty well—looking at this as an opportunity to lose some weight, grow more hair, sort of like an all inclusive resort. Think about it—no cooking, no dog, no kids, no spouse, no laundry, no cleaning, your own TV, your own PC, meals delivered to your room . . .

A cruise would be better, but this will do.

I was actually looking into a fat farm just before the diagnosis and was trying to convince a friend to go with me. Her attitude was why should she spend $3K to go somewhere to be yelled at by a drill sergeant and be fed three artfully arranged snow peas on a plate for dinner. She in turn tried to convince me to go on a cruise with a chocolate midnight buffet. Well, now I get the stem cell spa treatment instead. I wonder if there is chocolate on the menu?

It would be an honor to be involved in any way. Just let me know. I think the world of your work and efforts and am always amazed at your ability to not only be as creative as you are, but also your project management skills as well as people mojo. Most of the rest of us would be lucky just to have strengths in any one of those areas.

You have my cell; if you need anything, holler. I will be shuttling between NYC and upstate NY for awhile. Then at some point in late May or early June, I'll be in Weill-Cornell Medical/NY Presbyterian for two and a half to three weeks, and then in a Fortieth Street studio for about one hundred days. It's basic but okay; the best part is a huge pool and sauna in the basement, along with racquetball courts and a gym, laundry. Unfortunately, I will only be able to use the laundry. Go figure. What can I do?

It might be awhile before I get Internet set up at the studio or the hospital, but I will try to check my e-mail from time to time.

*Love,*
*Olivia*

From: Olivia Chin (oliviac@yahoo.com)     Sent: 04/11/09 1:10 PM
To: Friendlist
Cc:
Subject: Tapas Bar

Dear Friends,

Mary and I just came back from Tufts Medical, Boston yesterday, where I had a consult with Dr. Ray Comenzo, amyloidosis expert. Well, if only I had known! Tufts has one very significant distinct advantage over any other stem cell hospital—it is smack in the middle of Boston's Chinatown! Dim sum is available one block away!

Just a quick update and some info. Please keep in mind that all dates and durations are approximate. Even the medical protocol is subject to change. Dr. Comenzo is suggesting a change to Dr. Niesvizky and Dr. Mark in the chemo treatment, so things really are still in a state of flux.

I am starting the stem cell collection early next week at Weill-Cornell Medical, a.k.a. New York Presbyterian Hospital, on an outpatient basis. I will be in the city for at least eight days. Did you know the engineer who invented the stem cell extraction machine was an engineer at IBM Owego? He had a child with leukemia.

My motto in life (which was on my whiteboard for many years at work) has been: "Fill what's empty. Empty what's full. Scratch where it itches." Well, disregarding the itchy rash I have had now for almost a year, the process for collecting stem cells is to drive the production of these cells in the bone marrow sky high with meds, so much so that they pour out into your bloodstream, where they are collected by this machine which is somewhat similar to dialysis. (Empty what's full).

I hope to be able to come home for Mother's Day for a few days. Then the current plans are to start the stem cell transplant. This is where one gets high dose chemo to kill everything off, and they put your own stem cells back in and, hopefully, they graft and regenerate. (Fill what's empty). This is a two and a half to three-week process in the hospital. This will be done at Cornell Med. I get released when my immune gets back to a minimum level where the clean-room environment at the hospital is no longer needed.

Then the plan is to stay in NYC for ninety to one hundred days afterward. There are numerous doctors' visits, tests, and there are risks due to the compromised immune system that make it such that being in Owego does not make sense. Wai is going to take care of me for the first two to three weeks after discharge from the hospital. I will stay at the NYC studio we now have access to (thank you Helene!) followed by Louise (my fairy Godmother) for one to two weeks. Mary Nielsen will be at our house in Owego, taking care of Katie and Elizabeth. I hope to be strong enough after four to five weeks to fend for myself in NYC. When school lets out in late June, the kids will go to Michele for two weeks so she can reach canonization while living (she has four kids of her own). Then, I am hoping to ping on all of you who can to help with my kids during the day, since Wai and Mary have to work, I will be gone, and school is out. Those of you working parents with kids at home for the summer, perhaps you can connect with Wai and we can contribute to your childcare costs and share? (Basically, we run out of plans and will need to punt by mid-July for childcare). I am hoping my brother might be able to come by mid-July and help for a few weeks. Donna and Marcia Blowney-Toda, both neighbors, are going to help my mother. Cindy Ellen Stevens has graciously taken on potential care of Mambo, our irascible pup, when Wai is in NYC. Michael Blowney, Marcia's son, is there to help in NYC as well. The rest of you are on call. If Wai has to go to NYC without the kids to help me, I told him that besides my mom (who is ninety, enough said), I know I can count on you all to take the kids. Thank you all!

The actual results of the transplant will not be clear until ninety days after the transplant. The statistics for surviving the transplant itself are excellent; however the overall long-term outlook is rather grim. Basically, the life expectancy after five years sucks. However, Dr. Comenzo is the man to go to after the transplant to see what clinical trials might be available. I plan however to be around to fill your e-mail in baskets for quite some time. I know what the odds are, and I plan to beat all the odds. By a wide margin. That's it. There is no other alternative. Make sure you plan to play kickball with me when we are all in wheelchairs. I'll bet you my wheelchair will outrun yours. (Because Wai will monkey with the gear ratio so mine will take off like a rocket).

I may not be in touch for awhile, between still having to get e-mail set up in NYC and possibly just fatigue. If you have questions, please e-mail Mary Nielsen (on distribution of this e-mail).

Please don't send anything: no flowers, no fruit, no gifts, no massage therapists or Chippendale dancers, etc. There are a lot of restrictions due to the immune system, but cards or notes would be nice. (Gift cards and bank notes, that is. JUST KIDDING!).

Here is a laugh for the day: Last night, I came home from Boston with Mary. Mary heads for bed, the kids get hugged and go to bed, Wai and I sit down to talk. Wai wants to know what I found out and how the trip went. So I spill the data, including the dismal five—and ten-year survival rates. We get sad and teary, and he goes into that shutdown, limbo-land mode. Then I tell him about the trip and the food, and I get to the part about dinner at the tapas bar. He perks up, gets interested, and keeps asking me how we enjoyed the tapas bar. I said the tapas were pretty good, not great, the wine and cocktail were nice. The questions go back and forth until I start thinking his interest in tapas are rather unusual. Finally he says something like: "So did you really enjoy the topless bar?"

Love,
Olivia

From: Olivia Chin (<u>oliviac@yahoo.com</u>)    Sent: 04/21/2009 9:28 PM
To: "Nick You"
Cc:
Subject: Woman in Your Life

Dear Nicky,

I guess I'll meet P****a this summer. While I question the wisdom of
your decision to bring her to our mother's house when you come to
play with Katie and Elizabeth, I wish you luck. My opinion of bringing
new loved ones into the family fold is akin to watching a shark feeding
frenzy. On the other hand, since our family is more subdued, and we tend
to refrain from showing our feelings, perhaps we'll just appear as a polite
circle of buzzards pecking at the fresh victim, drawing blood. Just consider
yourself lucky that you do not have a posse of siblings!

Your girlfriends need to have all three Bs in order to pass my muster:
beauty, brains, and breeding. However, in order to pass Mom's muster, she
has to be a younger clone of Mom, except it can't be too obvious.

Anyway, you said that the man-cheese was mean and wicked. I failed to
share the woman-flower, which is just plain mean. Enjoy!

*Love,*
*Olivia*

## Women Are Like Flowers

*I met a woman today who was seventy-nine. She was slim, trim, and stylish. She sported a full head of beautiful white hair, which bobbed in the breeze. It occurred to me that she was like a flower, still in bloom, still beautiful. And then, the analogy between women and flowers blossomed.*

*Some women are like orchids or birds of paradise. They are exotic and elegant, ever so poised and almost extravagant in style. They do not wilt, they do not wane—they appear the same, even over time. They remain wise over the ages. Beautiful as a single bloom, these flowers are best displayed singly, to flaunt their independent character and beauty. These women eat sashimi and tapas. For dessert, they will enjoy passion fruit sorbet or tiramisu.*

*I love to look at cultivated long-stemmed roses. They are artificially beautiful. Their expensive and delicious perfume permeates a room. These flowers are stunning in their fresh youth, but they do not always age well. When they wilt, they droop, and their petals wrinkle at times. The thorns that are barely visible in their time of blooming glory become more prominent as they age. They detest being in the presence of other flowers, preferring to be grouped only with uncontested clumps of greens. When these women enter a room, not only do men's heads turn, they also turn into drooling fools. These women wear beautiful clothes with beautiful jewels, their hair well coiffed, their long-legged, tanned stems aglow. Just as roses are high maintenance, requiring trimming often, so are these women. They have never been seen to eat; they nibble vegetarian crudités. They may be seen with a petit four or a berry pavlova on their plate, but nobody has ever seen it touch their laquered lips.*

*A friend loves carnations. Slightly tacky, they last forever. They are dressed in outrageous colours that are never seen in nature. They are gaudy and trendy and fun. They can move their heads with attitude, blooms bobbing. They look lovely in lively groups. You can never get these women to shut up; they are always talking, laughing, and having a good time. They eat ribs with their hands and lick the tips of their fingers afterward. Then they demolish pecan pies or coconut layer cake for dessert.*

*Then there are the dandelions. They are not stunning, yet they can be beautiful. These tenacious flowers are so strong, they can overcome anything. They are well* grounded. Facing adverse conditions, they thrive. These flowers multiply quickly. These women are always surrounded by children, grandchildren, nieces and nephews, parents, aunts, uncles, and cousins. These women are plain and simple. However, they are always there to support you in times of need. These women eat hamburgers and fries followed by apple pie or blackberry cobbler for dessert.

I love to wander amongst wildflowers. Dancing in the wind, they are carefree. They love being outdoors in the sun. They sow their seeds with wild abandon. Their natural beauty is pure. When trapped in a vase, they cease to flourish. They live life fully and simply. These women enjoy being outdoors at lakeside cottages, toasting marshmallows at bonfires at night. They eat roasted beets with wild greens and goat cheese. They have been seen to enjoy granola yogurt smoothies for breakfast and chunky monkey ice cream for dessert.

Then there are the morning glories. I have planted these flowers, beguiled by their simple appearance, seemingly delicate beauty and allure, only to wrestle with clingy vines that can smother all signs of life. The vines are so persistent that removing them is almost an impossible mission. They grow with incredible abandon, using other plants as means of support. They kill as they assimilate. Morning glory women are so needy; they will eat up their girlfriends and destroy their mates. They will eat anything and suck the life force out of the remaining shards. Their appetite and neediness are voracious.

Last, there are moonflowers. If you are ever lucky enough to see these in bloom, you will have witnessed absolute beauty. These huge flowers blossom in the moonlight, as if they were opening their throats and singing their glorious song just for themselves. Not caring if others are there to enjoy or admire their beauty, they enjoy their inner secrets by themselves. They are plain by day, spectacular at night. These women are comfortable and secure with themselves. They revel in the community of women. These women eat heaping bowls of pasta, ratatouille, grilled rosemary chicken, and other natural foods to nourish their souls and bodies. They eat chocolate brownies and strawberry shortcake and mint chip ice cream cones for dessert.

I think I am a hybrid, a mutant combination of wildflower and orchid, with a hope of morphing into a moonflower. I eat like a morning glory. What about you?

From: Felicia@aol.com          Sent: 04/17/09 7:10 PM
To: Olivia
Cc:
Subject: None

Dear Olivia,

I just read your e-mail, and I am happy that you are doing well. Would you be kind enough to take my name off your addressee list? Thank you.

I wish you much success.

Felicia

From: WaiCh                                    Sent: 04/28/09 11:11 AM
To: Olivia
Cc:
Subject: Forwarding memo
FYI.
Wai

**From:** Hewson, Marillyn A
**Sent:** Monday, April 27, 2009 3:00 PM
**Subject:** Reduction in Force, May 2009

# *Memorandum*

DATE: April 27, 2009

TO: Lockheed Martin Systems Integration—Owego Employees

FROM: Marillyn Hewson, President

SUBJECT: Reduction in Force, May 2009

In response to a downturn in business conditions and recent announcements by the Secretary of Defense, we have completed an extensive review of current staffing needs and determined a reduction of approximately 225 positions is needed now, and a further reduction will likely be necessary in the months ahead as the Department of Defense budget is finalized.

The impact of this workforce reduction is not limited to any one program and will affect the entire enterprise, in both direct and indirect positions. Multiple external factors make this reduction necessary: uncertainty around the FY10 budget; the recommendation from the Secretary of Defense to cancel the VH-71 Presidential Helicopter program and to terminate the acquisition of the Air Force Combat Search and Rescue (CSAR-X) aircraft; delays in planned work for our postal customers; and other programs that have been delayed or cancelled.

Employees affected by the reduction in force will be notified in mid-May. To ease the transition from the business, affected employees will be eligible for severance benefits and other employment assistance. Meetings will be held with these employees to discuss opportunities in other Lockheed Martin businesses, outplacement services, and benefits continuation. The leadership team has been actively engaged in trying to reduce the need for job losses by aggressively pursuing work-share at other Lockheed Martin locations and reducing discretionary costs. These efforts have mitigated the need for more significant reductions at this time.

While we are taking these steps to maintain our business competitiveness and viability, we have preserved our funding for new business pursuits. We will focus on our core markets in rotary wing, modernization, and sustainment, where we see opportunities for growth. We'll also continue to pursue adjacent market opportunities, such as ground vehicles, evidenced by our recent win of the Joint Light Tactical Vehicle (JLTV) technology development contract. We also see growing interest in the international marketplace for our products and capabilities, and we are strategically addressing those opportunities.

As we move forward, I will continue to keep you informed. My intent is to ensure that you get the information that you need from me and your leadership team in a timely manner. If you have questions, please contact your management team or me.

Despite the recent setbacks and economic conditions our company is facing, we remain a strong business, with a very talented, dedicated team. We will focus on continued outstanding performance for our customers, and on pursuing opportunities to grow the business.

Thank you for your continued dedication and commitment to our business success.

From: Olivia Chin (oliviac@yahoo.com)     Sent: 05/06/09 11:10 PM
To: Friendlist
Cc:
Subject: All-Inclusive Resort Check-In Tomorrow

Dear Friends,

I have been down in NYC for the last ten days without a PC or Internet
connection until last night. WITHDRAWAL!!! It's a good thing this
city has so many wonderful distractions because it is amazing how PCs
have become a part of our lives. Can you imagine living without your
microwave, your PC, or cell phone? All I can say about my being without
a PC here is that NYC is a far, far better place because of it. I have been
promoting the Olivia Financial Stimulus Package. For the last ten days, I
have been shopping, eating, and running back and forth from the hospital,
but mostly shopping and eating.

A quick update. After self-injections of neupogen to promote stem cell
growth, I had my stem cells collected Monday and Tuesday. I do not
understand how people can give themselves shots. By Monday night,
the syringe needles were bending as I hyperventilated! I think my body
was fighting back! (No way, sister, are you putting that @#$&!! in me
again!)

I am checking into NY Presbyterian Hospital tomorrow morning to start
the stem cell infusion/transplant. I am considering this as checking into an
all-inclusive weight loss resort, except I'm told the food is extraordinarily
bad, and there are no free margaritas. The stay lasts two to three weeks.
The room is on the top floor of a tower, hopefully with great views of
the East River. Private room, filtered airflow, restricted visitors, and when
the immune really tanks, well, let's just say it'll be like Rapunzel in the
tower, only minus the hair.

Wai and the kids came down last weekend. The nurse thought it would
help the kids see part of the process, and the social worker thought it
would help them see the unit. They were allowed to see the machine in
action, collecting my stem cells, and they went for a quick visit of the stem
cell transplant unit. Katie hates anything to do with the insides of bodies.

I have these tubes hanging out of my upper chest, a tunneled catheter (resistance is futile!). When Katie saw the tubes getting connected to the pheresis (collection) machine, the nurse was worried she was going to pass out! The nurse, Inja, was still chuckling yesterday over Katie's facial expressions. It was hard to say good-bye to the kids on Monday. I was able to keep it together, but as I saw Elizabeth leaving the room, Inja raced to get a box of tissues. I honked long and loud. Then Dr. Mark, my stem cell transplant doctor came by, and then left promptly only to return with the loaner of his personal Nintendo DS!

Dr. Niesvizky is the senior physician, clinical director et al, and Dr. Mark is a younger physician who handles all the autologous stem cell patients and amyloid patients. Thanks to these two, I had another bone marrow sample taken about two weeks ago. I am not sure what prompted Dr. Niesvizky to feel that the test needed to be repeated. Experience? Intuition? In any event, when asked to repeat this rather unpleasant test, I said that the anal part of me would be pleased to have symmetrical holes in my derrière. After the stem cell transplant is over and the immune system is recovered, I will probably start chemo, hopefully at home.

Wai has been wonderful. He has been caring but not smothering. He is quiet and just checks on me once in awhile. We have always run our lives in a very independent manner. For the first time ever, he has been bringing me café lattes and a newspaper in the morning. Life is good.

I do not know if I will have access to e-mail for the next two to three weeks. I will have my cell phone with me. Please do not feel insulted if I do not return your calls at times. I understand this resort can really work you hard at times. If you just want a quick update, please e-mail Mary. Mary is a close friend who is staying at our house for now, helping out. Thanks to everyone for all the help, calls, and support. The prayers and good vibes are working.

*Love,*
*Olivia*

# PRE-STEM CELL TRANSPLANT: MEDICAL PERSPECTIVE

The term *stem cell* hearkens the thorny ethical debate of the proper treatment and care of human embryos. These stem cells are derived from the earliest stages of human development and theoretically can give rise to any other kind of cell or organ tissue type in the body. Not all stem cells are the same, however. The hematopoietic stem cells (HPCs) used in hematopoietic (bone marrow) stem cell transplants, for instance, are not taken from an embryonic source, but are instead harvested from an adult. These particular stem cells can give rise to elements of the bone marrow and bloodstream, (platelets, red and white blood cells), but not to a new liver. HPCs used to be collected through a series of bone marrow biopsies performed in an operating room setting. Now we use chemicals to convince the HPCs staying in the bone marrow space to come out into the peripheral bloodstream in a process called *mobilization* so that they can be collected via a machine. We can use the peripheral blood stem cells (PBSCs) then for a transplant.

There are several different kind of transplants used for the treatment of hematologic diseases, but they break down into two major types based on the source of stem cells: 1) autologous, and 2) allogeneic. Autologous stem cell transplants involve the collection from and infusion of stem cells into the same person, i.e., the donor and recipient are the same. The purpose of the HPCs in the autologous transplant is not to simply give back stem cells; rather, it allows the patient to receive a very high dose of chemotherapy without running a high risk of death of prolonged marrow failure related to the chemotherapy itself. The infusion of the HPCs immediately following the chemotherapy allows the rapid recovery of bone marrow populations and function, thus exposing the disease (be it myeloma, lymphoma, etc.) to the chemotherapy, but allowing the patient to survive the exposure as well. For this reason, autologous stem cell transplants are also correctly termed *high-dose chemotherapy with stem cell rescue*.

The figure below illustrates the concept of the autologous stem cell transplant. Chemotherapy is first infused, followed by the stem cells about two days later. The blood counts then begin to drop in response to the chemotherapy. The stem cells then begin to populate the bone marrow and the blood counts recover (this is called *engraftment*). The period between the drop in blood counts and engraftment is called the nadir. The nadir is the most dangerous time during the transplant, where the white cell, red cell, and platelet counts are low, and the patient is at risk for infection and usually needs blood transfusions. Without the stem cell support, the nadir period would be very long, thus exposing the patient to a greater time of risk.

In contrast to the autologous stem cell transplant, where the primary purpose of the procedure is give high-dose chemotherapy safely, an allogeneic transplant involves the use of stem cells obtained from a different person to infuse into the donor. A major goal of the allogeneic transplant is to harness the immune system of the donor to attack the malignant cells in the recipient—this is called the *graft versus tumor effect*. Of course, inherent in this proposition is the possibility that the donor cells will start attacking the recipient's body in addition to the tumor—this is called *graft versus host disease* (GVHD). GVHD makes allogeneic stem cell transplantation a bit more risky, and even with proper immunosuppressive drug manipulation, the overall mortality rate hovers in the 15 percent range. For comparison, the risk of death with an autologous stem cell transplant, where GVHD is not a factor, is approximately 1 percent. For the rest of this section, we will focus only on autologous stem cell transplant, which is what Olivia went through.

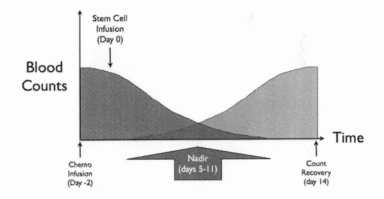

Prior to transplant, all patients undergo an intense body check: pulmonary function testing, twenty-four-hour urine collection for creatinine clearance, dental screening, donor screening blood tests, bone marrow biopsy, plain sinus X-ray, and chest X-ray. The purpose of the testing is to ensure that the patient will be able to withstand the rigors of the procedure and high-dose chemotherapy.

The nuts and bolts of the process of stem cell mobilization, collection, and storage follows. There are many different techniques to mobilize stem cells to come out of the bone marrow and circulate in the bloodstream, but one of the most common ways is to use a cytokine (cytokine = a chemical signal that the body makes to tell cells to behave in a certain fashion) called neupogen (a.k.a. filgastrim, G-CSF, granulocyte colony stimulating factor). The patient self-injects neupogen subcutaneously on a nightly basis for four nights. On the day before, or morning of, the start of stem cell collection, a catheter is placed via tunneling underneath the skin into a large blood vessel to allow for the pheresis procedure. This catheter has two ports, one to allow blood exit and the other to allow entry, and usually remains in place throughout the course of the stem cell transplant. After four doses of neupogen, the patient undergoes the pheresis procedure to collect stem cells. The pheresis machine looks very much like a dialysis machine; blood exits the body through the catheter, enters the machine, gets processed, returns from the machine through the catheter, and then back into the patient. Inside the machine, the blood is spun in a centrifuge and separated according to density. The layer in which the white blood cells (including stem cells) reside is taken off, and the rest is given back to the patient. Inside the machine, a chemical called citrate is used to prevent blood clotting. Some persons have a reaction to this, as the citrate can leech calcium. The reaction usually consists of facial tingling or hand twitching and is addressed promptly with infusion of intravenous calcium. Most patients do not experience any reaction at all; in fact, I often tell patients that the most frequent side effect is boredom because a day of stem cell collection usually takes between four to five hours.

Once the collection is done for the day, the patient goes home. The stem cell lab counts the number of cells collected and determines if another day of collection is needed to achieve the goal (usually the goal is to collect enough stem cells to support two transplants). If another day of collection is needed, the patient gets a phone call, directing her to inject another dose of neupogen that night and come in the next day to collect again. Once the goal number of stem cells is achieved, we arrange for hospital admission for transplant. Any leftover cells are frozen and stored at very low temperature to allow for their potential use in the future via cryopreservation.

For stem cell transplantation, the patient is admitted to a hospital private room under negative air pressure isolation and hepa filtering. Upon admission, chemotherapy will be given usually in split doses over several days. After chemotherapy, the stem cells are infused through the pheresis catheter, in much the same manner as a standard blood transfusion. Then, we wait. In most cases, no side effects appear for about three to four days after chemotherapy. After this period, the patient enters the nadir, where the blood counts drop. There is a period anywhere from six to fifteen days where her blood counts would be very low and there is high susceptibility to infection. We typically give prophylactic antibiotics, but there is still a risk of fever and severe blood infections. Most people also require red blood cell and platelet transfusion support so that no complications of severe anemia (shortness of breath, headache, weakness) or low platelet count (bleeding) occur. Most people also lose their hair at this time. Other less frequent complications that may occur are diarrhea, mouth sores, and nausea—fortunately, these are all temporary. All patients recover the blood counts, but normally feel weak for up to three months. Most patients also lose their appetite and on average lose ten to fifteen pounds during the transplant period. All patients also receive prophylactic medicines to take at home, including acyclovir, to prevent late-occurring infections.

The transplant recovery process takes up to one year, but most symptoms are resolved within the first one hundred days after the stem cell infusion. The biggest persistent side effect is fatigue. Most people have a tough time getting off the couch for the first couple of weeks after they get home. Some can get winded just getting up to go the bathroom and back! Within a few weeks, however, energy starts to seep back in. People begin to eat more, get out more, and are able to do more tasks. Usually by eight weeks, most are completely independent. The risk of infection remains high, however, since more time is needed for the immune system to recover. Advice is given to avoid large groups of people (something as simple as being near an aberrant cough or sneeze from another person can lead to a hospital admission) and also to avoid certain uncooked or unprocessed foods. This lasts for about one hundred days, at which point the patient usually feels well enough to go back to work.

Most people lose some immunity memory to prior vaccinations. At one year, titers to old vaccines are rechecked and revaccination is performed as needed.

The average time after a transplant until there is new progression of the original disease varies. For myeloma it ranges between two to three years. For Hodgkin lymphoma, autologous transplantation can be curative. Given that myeloma and amyloid are not cured by transplant, certain techniques to prolong this time of disease stability post-transplant are under investigation. This will be the subject of the next section.

Transplant is definitely NOT for everyone. Given that it can be a tough procedure to get through, the very elderly (> eighty years old) or the very frail are not usually good candidates, especially if the disease is not curable. For these patients, continued chemotherapy is usually a better option. Some persons eligible for transplant actually tolerate and prefer the continuous chemotherapy and choose to not undergo the transplant or wait for a time when the chemotherapy stops working. This is also a reasonable option, as, in the case of myeloma, there is no difference in overall survival whether the transplant is done early or later in the clinical course.

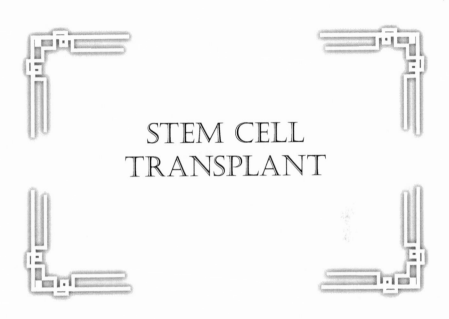

# STEM CELL
# TRANSPLANT

From: Olivia Chin (oliviac@yahoo.com)    Sent: 05/09/09 10:18 AM
To: Friendlist
Cc:
Subject: All-Inclusive Resort

Dear Friends,

Hi everyone!

I checked into the hospital on Thursday. I got two high doses of chemo (Melphalan) on Thursday and Friday... My stem cells, which were collected earlier this week, will return to me on Monday. Right now, all is well, but I understand the descent will start on Tuesday or Wednesday. It takes approximately ten days for the stem cells to graft and grow, so it'll only be a short while hopefully until my immune system starts rebuilding. I am still a little sore—a side effect of the neupogen injections.

If you remember, I have these ports coming out of my upper chest, the tunneled catheter. This was very uncomfortable initially, but I am feeling it less now. It only took a day to understand the benefits of this catheter. Almost everything that needs to go in or come out (medications, chemo, stem cells, blood tests, etc.) is done via these ports, and it is totally painless.

While able to receive e-mails, I will no longer be able to send them until further tinkering with our PC. You are getting this via Wai. He has been carting the laptop out of the hospital and sending them via an external Internet link. But Wai will be heading back to Owego for the next two weeks. I am going to miss getting café lattes and the NY Times! Wai has been so sweet. It's nice being spoiled! I may be spoiled, but I am also bored, so all the nurses and aides are now sporting earrings. Yup. I came here with one light bag of clothes and two heavy bags of beads! I am making jewelry as a way to pass the time. By the time I get out of here, I should be able to open a jewelry shop (unless I keep giving it all away). Dr. Mark teased me about having to extend my stay here.

BTW, there is one very disturbing issue with this resort. The brochure advertised views of the East River or the Manhattan skyline. My room, however, is called "Pebble Beach" by the resort staff, because the view consists of several tons of pebbles on a rooftop. No river. No skyline. No Zen-inspired raking of pebbles. In fact, this room is on one of the highest floors of the hospital, and I am puzzled how a green soda bottle ended up on Pebble Beach. I tried the windows and found them firmly screwed shut. Does that means there will be no nude sunbathing on the rooftop?

Love,
Olivia

From: Olivia Chin (oliviac@yahoo.com)    Sent: 05/11/09 11:38 AM
To: Friendlist
Cc:
Subject: Day Zero at Pebble Beach

Dear Friends,

Today is Day Zero for me. Day Zero is how one refers to the day you get your stem cells back. I asked one of the nurses why it is called Day Zero, and she said it is the beginning of a new life. It didn't seem right to tell her I thought it referred to a nuclear wipe out! The actual event was rather . . . uneventful. A bag of my stem cells was infused into me via the port, just like the chemo.

I do need to share with you how incredible everyone is here. Dr. Mark, as the stem cell transplant physician, stops by every working day. He even lent me his Nintendo DS! He told me Dr. Niesvizky would be doing the educational rounds next week. This week it is up to Dr. S, who came in today with the usual entourage of medical students. He introduced himself as the clinical director of the stem cell facility. He is most entertaining!

The first nurse I had, Cathy, will forever be remembered as an absolute angel. It turns out we have the same birthday—yesterday! When she found out I was going to be by myself on my birthday, which also coincided with Mother's Day, she took some time out from her busy life and brought me a card and this incredibly rich and delicious dark chocolate ganache cake. Heaven!

The cleaning lady, Ruby, noticed while she was wiping down the doorknobs with bleach that I was cold. Without asking, she went and got an extra blanket, and then she tucked me in like a baby. She really touched me with her gentle gesture.

One of the nurse aides noticed that I moved to the sleeper couch. She asked me if I was a light sleeper. I told her I usually could sleep through an earthquake, but that the hospital bed anti-bedsore feature was keeping me up. She found time after doing her rounds to read the manual on the hospital bed. She came back, pushed some buttons, frowned, pushed some more buttons, and frowned some more. She left and returned some time after. She went to check out other beds! She determined the bed I had was defective, and it was making an unusual loud, grinding noise. She put the order in for another bed to be brought in the morning.

This is some resort!

*Love,*
*Olivia*

From: Olivia Chin (oliviac@yahoo.com)     Sent: 05/15/09 3:38 AM
To: Friendlist
Cc:
Subject: Day Four at Pebble Beach

Dear Friends,

I am starting to feel tired. My body doesn't feel like mine. My sense of taste is very off. I take a shower every morning, but today I just couldn't get myself going. Things got better after that first cup of java! That cup of joe, however, is beginning to taste weird. Food does not taste that good. (Did I actually say that?)

A venture out of my room to get a Doppler ultrasound (one of the physicians was worried about DVTs) was exhausting. While waiting for someone to wheel me back to my room, I was breathing so heavily into my face mask after the procedure that the other patients also waiting for their "chauffeurs" started yelling, "Lady in distress!" I didn't even realize they were referring to me!

Some of you have asked me what I do. Mainly I sleep. But here is a summary of my day:

Vitals early in the morning
Gargle with special mouthwash
Blood draw early in the morning
Shower and wash up
Insulin shot
*Breakfast & Yogurt*
Room cleaning and linen change
Meds
Medical student and physician rounds
Joke around with Dr. S or Dr. Niesvizky
Nap
Read
Look at results from morning blood test
Make some jewelry
Call a friend

Read
Vitals
Gargle
Insulin shot
*Lunch & Yogurt*
Dr. Mark visit (I try not to sleep until he comes!)
Read
Nap
Make some jewelry or just sit up
Read
Vitals
Gargle
Insulin shot
*Dinner & Yogurt*
Meds
Read
Call Wai, talk to Katie and Elizabeth
Watch TV
Insulin shot
Sleep
Vitals
Gargle
Stay up for a few hours
*Eat several Italian lemon ices and a spoon of yogurt to throw off blood sugar
tests*
Sleep

I was told on the first day by the social worker that gargling might help minimize future mouth sores. Provided with this room were these two bottles of funky mouthwash. If all I have to do is gargle to avoid bad mouth sores, gargle and gargle I will. The yogurt is my personal attempt to avoid the side effects of antibiotics and chemo. It can't hurt.

Everything is starting to taste really bad. I noticed if I order tuna salad, the fishiness of the tuna masks the nasty taste. Crackers with peanut butter are all I can manage sometimes.

I never thought I could lose interest in food. (Invasion of the body snatchers!)

Love,
Olivia

PS: Four or more shots a day. I am a human pincushion!

From: Olivia Chin (oliviac@yahoo.com)     Sent: 05/19/09 4:21 PM
To: Friendlist
Cc:
Subject: Fatigue and Food Fantasies


Hi.


This is the first time in days since I've had the strength to get the PC
out of the bag. I am sooo tired! You know it's bad when you need to
pee, the bathroom is not ten feet from your bed, and you are seriously
considering letting loose in the bed and ringing the nurse afterward.
Getting out of bed is hard. Eating is hard. Swallowing those pills is hard.
Taking a morning shower takes a few hours.

Thank you all for your calls, help, wishes, cards, and more. It means so
much more than you will ever know. Thank you also with helping my
family—just knowing you are there to help is such a comfort. Please
don't get mad at me if I do not answer your calls, I am too wiped out.
Your voicemails bring great joy.

Dr. Niesvizky and Dr. Mark also bring great joy when they do their
daily rounds. I am so happy to see them, I feel like The Great Pumpkin.
I cannot subdue the smile that bubbles up when they stop by. I am so
lucky to have these men in my life.

I haven't been out of this room since Monday 5/11/09. Until today, I'm
not sure I could have anyway—I am dealing with a level of fatigue that
is beyond numbing. I am near the nadir of my treatment. Lost about
fifteen pounds. A lot of time is spent in bed, lying down, sleeping, or just
staring at the ceiling. Even TV is too much to bear at times. The doctors
expect me to get worse yet, but I know better. I am on the mend. Do
you know how I can tell?

Yesterday, early in the morning, I finally got hungry for the first time.
I dreamt about my Godmother Louise's stuffed artichokes. I craved a
perfect summer tomato. I lusted for a perfect slice of semolina bread
with Helene and Dennis's tamaroasalata. I fantasized about roasted beet
salad with arugula and goat cheese. I longed for a really rich, creamy

vegetable korma. I am having immoral thoughts about my mother's pork dumplings. Don't even stop to think about what I would do for a glass of chilled Gewurztraminer.

Do you think I should tell the doctors they can stop the anti-nausea meds now?

*Love,*
*Olivia*

From: Olivia Chin (oliviac@yahoo.com)    Sent: 05/19/2009 8:18 PM
To: "Nick You"
Cc:
Subject: RE: Dumplings

Dear Nicky,

I am sorry to inform you that you do not have the exclusive on food fantasies!

It would appear obvious that our obsessions with food are genetic. Katie, though, has an amazing set of taste buds, and she loves good food. I remember her list for suggested lunch items as we prepared for Kindergarten; it included king crab legs, shrimp, and lobster. My list consisted of carrot sticks, PB&J on whole wheat bread, and cheese and crackers. So she is living proof of the impact of family environment. I cannot speak for Elizabeth's rather simple tastes in food, except to say that Wai stayed at home for her early years, shortly after her adoption.

You asked about Wai and marriage. Coming from the one who is breaking up with Number Three, I do not know if that makes you a fool or an expert. Speaking of Wai, I told him how much he meant to me. Being apart for several weeks is not new to us. However, being apart while one of us is undergoing a stem cell transplant is quite the novel experience. I had plenty of time to think about relationships with family and friends. So I told him that between work and kids and volunteer efforts and Mom and the dog and the house and the yard, our relationship had become overrun by events. And that once I am home, this situation needs to change. I want more than what we have had in many years. I want more than collaborating on sharing tasks just to keep afloat with clean clothes, food on the table, and kids' activities. I want more in what time I have left. We all deserve more.

I also gave him an out. Dealing with this disease until now has been a picnic compared to what may be coming ahead. I have had too many friends with cancer whose significant other ditched them in their times of dire need. So I told Wai that if he cannot deal with my future—which is not the same as will not—that he could walk away, no hard feelings. I don't want him to endure that which he will come to resent or hate. He has never been able to deal with illness well.

He says he is here to stay.

I am really proud of my family right now. Wai has risen to the occasion. Between taking care of me, taking care of the kids, and dealing with the unusual stress factors at work, he has been there for everyone. I am concerned. The recent decisions with the new administration are going to result in huge layoffs in Owego—the rumors are one out of five will be let go. Wai and I are concerned about medical insurance. If he gets laid off, we know that we have squirreled away enough so that we can stay in the house and eat. The major issue would be medical insurance.

The kids have held up really well. They understand what is happening. We explained to them that the treatment will allow me to live longer and spend more time with them. We also asked them to help. When I was at home, they handled a lot of chores. Before I left, they seemed preoccupied with their hair, practicing on each other's long hair, making braids, buns, and ponytails. I learned that these sessions were their preparation for dance competitions. Their report cards are excellent; it looks like all As are coming up.

Love,
Olivia

From: WaiCh                                    Sent: 05/20/09 10:01 AM
To: Olivia
Cc:
Subject: Forwarding memo

FYI.

Wai

DATE: May 19, 2009

TO: Lockheed Martin Systems Integration—Owego Employees

FROM: Marillyn Hewson, President

SUBJECT: Reduction in Force—Notification

Today we notified approximately 130 of our colleagues that they would
no longer have employment with the company after 90 days of continued
pay and benefits. Due to attrition, movement of employees to other
Lockheed Martin companies, and evolving workload changes, the actual
number of affected employees is less than the projected 225 reductions
announced on April 27.

We have initiated procedures in compliance with the Workers Adjustment
Retraining Notification (WARN) process, which contains both federal
and state provisions. WARN affords continued pay and benefits for 90
days from the day of notification of loss of employment, and is required
by law in New York for a planned reduction of 250 or more positions. We
initiated the WARN process since we do anticipate a further reduction
in force in the near future, for which the aggregate reduction will be
greater than 250.

To help ease the transition from the business, affected employees will
be eligible for severance benefits. A joint Lockheed Martin and New
York Department of Labor team will conduct informational meetings
for affected employees to discuss how to search for opportunities in
other Lockheed Martin businesses and provide information about

outplacement services, benefits continuation, and general employment assistance. Employees at offsite locations will be provided access to the same resources. More information, including frequently asked questions regarding the reduction in force, will be available on Passport under the "Frequently Used Links" section of MyOwego, or by clicking here.

Since my first announcement on April 6, following Secretary of Defense Gates' budget recommendations, we have worked steadfastly to mitigate the impact to jobs. Unfortunately, continued pressure exerted on the VH-71 Presidential Helicopter program through the budgetary process and corresponding customer direction to stop work, will make it difficult to hold our current staffing levels.

Our colleagues who have been affected by this current reduction will continue to be valued members of our team throughout the 90-day WARN period. I ask you to support them as teammates, as we provide resources to help ease their transition in the months ahead.

From: Olivia Chin (oliviac@yahoo.com)     Sent: 05/20/09 7:35 PM
To: Friendlist
Cc:
Subject: Top Ten Preparation Tips for This Resort
    and Special Announcement

Hi everyone!

Interest in food I found out is not the same as eating with gusto. I had three small sores in my mouth, which I think resulted from biting myself while in that nebulous transition state between being awake and drifting off to slumber land. Other than being curiously flat, my stomach is about the same as always. The medicinal and metallic taste in my mouth seems to have the most impact when eating tomatoes and ... chocolate! When I realized I could not enjoy chocolate, conspiracy theories started forming. This is just not right! Downright un-American!

My hair fell out. It doesn't just drift off. It comes out in humongous clumps. I clogged the drain in the shower. When I got my glasses back on while showering to see why I was standing in a few inches of water, I thought a small black Lab puppy had somehow sneaked into the bathroom. After I showered, I decided it would be best not to look into the mirror. I went back to bed, slept, only to wake up with a hair-covered pillow. In forty-eight hours, it was all gone. The doctors are teasing me about it—that it might come back curly or wavy. I don't care if it comes back orange and kinky—I JUST WANT SOME HAIR BACK!

In their infinite wisdom, the doctors decided I needed transfusions of platelets and red blood cells. My counts in both of these are low. Platelets help your blood clot. Red blood cells help bring oxygen to you. I definitely felt better afterward. So—go out there and donate blood! And those of you who are willing, go get the inside of your mouths swiped so they can figure out if you are a match to someone who needs stem cells! They can collect your stem cells in a relatively painless manner without boring into your bones. Go forth and save a life!

I am done. The soapbox tipped over.

In the last week or so, I have formulated my top ten tips for this all-inclusive resort. Here goes:

1) Cut your nails short. Really short. *Since they won't let me cut my nails due to the low platelet count, and I didn't pack nail clippers anyway, you really need to trim your nails before coming here. Make sure you cut those toenails, since it is difficult to gnaw them short. When I look at my feet, all I can think about is that creature from Lord of the Rings.*

2) Cut your hair off. *Not short. Off. My hair was cut into a short "do," but it hurt as it fell out and tangled on the pillowcase. Getting all my hair shaved off before it started falling off on it's own would have been less painful and would also have avoided the shock of seeing the huge clumps fall out.*

3) Bring something entertaining. *Thank goodness for those tons of beads Wai was cussing about when he hauled them in here. I am so glad I had something to do that was not too tiring, yet creative. The entire unit here has received earrings. Whether they want them or not is irrelevant!*

4) Bring some light reading. *The key word is "light." This is not the time to catch up on reading those ten-pound tomes of depressing Russian literature or great French works. War and Peace. The Red and Black. When the fatigue hits, the more serious reading material went by the wayside for me. Magazines, light novels, and newspapers were definitely easier to handle. Did I mention that the nurses and nurse aides here are so sweet? They buy me newspapers on their breaks.*

5) Pack some allowable snacks. *Wai brought me these hard lemon candies that taste wonderful; they hide the chemo taste. The lemon Italian ices that the hospital provides are also pretty good. I wish I had packed some of those oversized popsicles in plastic tubes.*

6) Gargle. *It could be that I just lucked out with minimal mouth sores, minimal nausea, and a short bout intestinal malaise, but I believe gargling from the first day every four to six hours made a difference. This was a tip from the social worker when I first checked in, on Day Minus Four.*

7) Eat yogurt. *Nobody said this would help, but between chemo and the antibiotics, I figured this could only help with keeping some bacterial fauna and flora going in my plumbing. The hospital provided me with three to four yogurts a day. I ate a spoonful at every meal (even those meals where all I could manage was peanut butter and a cracker) and another when I woke up in the wee hours of the morning. The day the intestinal malaise spiked was . . . a mess. I cried and cried. I hate this disease. I hate the feeling of total loss of control.*

8) Pack your cell phone charger. *I packed the cell phone charger, an MP3 player, and the charger for the MP3 player, a laptop, and the charger for the laptop, a pay-per-use cell phone, and the charger for the second cell phone. Whew!*

9) Drink lots of water. *Drink water like a camel. Nobody told me to do this, and I don't know if the doctors would agree. My thoughts on this are simply this: Your body now has a lot of toxic stuff in it, not to mention a few more gugabazillion dead cells than usual. Drinking water is one way to help cleanse your system, right? They won't allow you gin and tonics anyway. I normally drink eight to ten oversized glasses of water a day, so this was not hard to do. Getting out of bed to go to the bathroom often, however . . .*

10) Pack more underwear and pajamas than you can imagine. Pack some street clothes. *I knew before checking into this resort that laundry facilities were not available. I thought I was covered with four pajamas and a gazillion panties. I did not anticipate the sweating. I had to ask a single, straight guy, whom I just recently befriended, to do my laundry. He probably has never seen underwear so large! Oh the humiliation of it all! (Wai meet Michael, Michael this is Wai). If there is any room left in your baggage after you have packed your beads, your reading material, and all the electronic gear and chargers, massive quantities of underwear and PJs and slippers, pack some street clothes. One outfit or two. You will have the outfit you wore when you checked in, so at least you will not leave the hospital nude or in sleepwear. Although I spent most of the time in pajamas, there were some days when it made me feel better to be in regular clothing.*

And a grand finale with good news!

*Wai and Olivia Chin are delighted and excited to announce the newly born White Blood Cells. We are pleased to witness the slightest increase in Olivia's White Blood Cell count. Please join us in celebrating this most joyous and awaited occasion. Her stem cells engrafted and are very hard at work.*

*Love,*
*Olivia*

From: Olivia Chin (oliviac@yahoo.com)     Sent: 05/22/09 5:39 PM
To: Friendlist
Cc:
Subject: Upgraded Room with View

Dear Friends,

My morale has significantly improved. I have been whining to whoever will listen about the conditions at Pebble Beach. Upon check-in, Wai and I checked out the floor plan by the elevator, and we found an enormous room in this tower unit. Unfortunately, the patient in this room did not check out as early as planned, despite the positive energy waves I was sending that way along with Krishna chants. Well, it became available, and I moved in!

The nurses had to help me pack. I moved in and promptly napped. How am I ever going to function after discharge? I can hardly find the energy to shower and brush my teeth every day.

This room is incredible—about two to three times larger than the one at Pebble Beach. There are views of the Queensborough Bridge and the Manhattan skyline, the East River, Roosevelt Island, and the windows wrap around this corner room. It seems lately I wake up and stay up every night in the wee hours of the morning, so now I eat my lemon ice and spoonful of yogurt in a tall chair facing the bridge and spectacular skyline. I have been told this is one of the best rooms in the entire hospital.

One disturbing thing: the view of Roosevelt Island includes three tall smokestacks. There is this movie with Mel Gibson and Julia Roberts, where he keeps reverting to this view of the same three smoke stacks. He is somewhat deranged, and if I remember, there is a top floor of a hospital involved. Hmm . . .

Even more fun is the much-anticipated iPod coordinated event on Roosevelt Island. The nurses have told me I may have some staff members in my room when that occurs. They are going to somehow all synchronize taking vitals, taking blood, cleaning my catheter, etc. Let's party!

Love,
Olivia

From: Olivia Chin (oliviac@yahoo.com)    Sent: 05/25/09 11:22 AM
To: Friendlist
Cc:
Subject: Extended Stay in Upgraded Room

Hello everyone!

I was doing really well last week and then Thursday hit. I was to be discharged on Saturday, but the discharge has been moved to tomorrow, Tuesday. I had this teensy little fever, and it wiped me out! I slept for an entire day, only half awake when the nurses came to take vitals, which I vaguely recall doubled or tripled in number.

Wai came down to help me get to Hope Lodge, only to end up helping me in the hospital. So far, he has provided me with much joy: roast pork pernil with rice and beans and yucca, vegetable-steamed bao, rice congee . . . Oh—and his company, of course! I cannot begin to describe to you the level of fatigue. Mind numbing. Beyond mind numbing. So Wai's gifts of food from The Great Outside have been able to pierce the fatigue. Wai is my Prince Charming. I am, of course, Sleeping Beauty. Food is the kiss of love, yucca the awakening of the senses, congee the gruel of life, bao the elixir of health.

And the café lattes!

He has been enjoying this room as well. The view is spectacular. By day, you can watch people walking along the river and count the barges and tugboats. Sailboats with spinnakers unfurled glide by. Large cruisers motor by, leaving huge white wakes. By night, the skyline sparkles! The bridge looks like a dazzling diamond necklace draped over a dark velvet river. Traffic patterns on FDR Drive and the bridge are interesting to monitor as well. After I thoroughly trounced Wai playing Scrabble (with wiped down letter tiles), and when he heard I had to stay three more days in this room, he asked me what I did to cause my temperature to spike!

My WBC is back within normal range and has been for several days. Platelets and RBC are still low. This place is amazing—within a few hours of the fever, they had triple blood samples express-shipped out of here to some infectious disease lab. The doctors are hoping that all the cultures come back negative and that the fever is due to graft issues with stem cell production, a rather common condition. But in the meantime, they have sent three samples out, each sample in triplicate drawn from three different sites. An infectious disease doctor also came and checked me out, calling in over the weekend to check lab results.

Tomorrow, we leave here for Hope Lodge, a residence provided free to cancer patients, right in Manhattan. It is run by the American Cancer Society. After Hope Lodge, we will be staying at a studio until I can go home. You can reach me via my cell phone.

Did you who know about my two trips to Rochester, NY, the last two years, where I volunteer and work on these mega-balloon art exhibits run by Larry Moss? His work stems from his family's experience with cancer (check out www.balloonmanor.com). He plans to repeat his annual Halloween exhibit this fall in Rochester, but the plans for a gigantic balloon art exhibit are in the works for Madison Square Garden, with the beneficiary to be Hope Lodge! Larry has asked me if I will help give the opening tour. I'll be honored to do it, even if I have to crawl around on my hands and knees!

I will be in touch to keep you all updated. Your calls, messages, cards, and more have been a wonderful source of comfort.

Love,
Olivia

From: Olivia Chin (oliviac@yahoo.com)     Sent: 05/26/09 2:43 PM
To: Friendlist
Cc:
Subject: Discharge Today!

Hi!

*My bags are packed; I'm ready to go . . . Taxi's waiting . . .*

Late this morning, I was wheeled off to have the catheter removed. I
was given a choice: five shots of local anesthesia or none and a quick rip.
I asked the doctor what he would prefer; he said the quick rip was less
painful.

*Liar! Liar! Pants on fire!*

I will acquiesce and acknowledge that the rip was quick. It was not,
however, without pain. You know that feeling one has as one just tips
over the top of the first ascent on a roller coaster? That fear so great
no sound emits, and your mouth is wide open in a silent scream? Yup.
Mouth wide open, no scream, toes scrunched, fingers gripped, and tears
pouring. As I slowly regained control of myself, I looked at the physician
with hate and lightening bolts, and I asked him if he enjoyed S&M,
especially the S part. He stomped off, telling me to hold the cotton pad
down on the site.

*How to make friends and influence people.*

We're waiting for the pharmacist to deliver prescription medication—an
enormous list. Then we're off! As excited as I am, I am also scared of
leaving. What if someone sneezes on me? How am I going to cope?
What if something goes wrong? This hospital unit was so well run—if
I even turned my light on in the wee hours of the morning, someone
would pop in to see if I was all right. The hand-cleaning protocol was
so thorough and so well followed. How do I know my room at Hope
Lodge is clean? How am I going to get food? What if I run out of toilet
paper? I try to calm my fears. The social worker tells me reassuringly that
this fear is normal.

The next time you hear from me, I will be at Hope Lodge.

*Love,*
*Olivia*

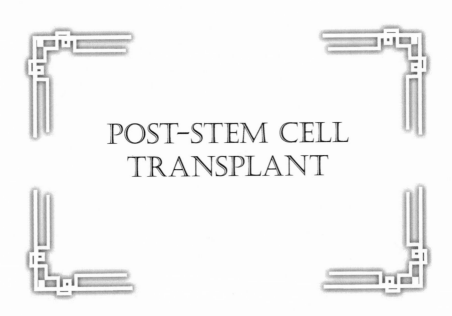

# POST–STEM CELL TRANSPLANT

Hi everyone!

I got out of the hospital last Tuesday. We were referred to Hope Lodge NYC, a truly amazing place. Hope Lodge is run by the American Cancer Society. It is a totally free residence for cancer patients and their caregivers. It is much more than a residence. They provide beautiful accommodations in the middle of Manhattan. In addition to sixty hotel-like rooms, there are laundry and kitchen facilities, quiet little reading nooks, as well as an enormous common area. The common area is beautifully appointed and quite upscale. It is divided in larger and smaller sitting areas, a game room, a library, a PC room, a Zen meditation room, a huge outside terrace, as well as another large kitchen. Everything here has been designed to make life easier for those either receiving treatment or recovering from treatment.

I am not usually sentimental, but I cried when I first saw this place. It is such a special feeling to know that there are sponsors who help design, build, and then maintain such incredible places. Just to give you an idea of the financial impact of some treatments, my stem cell process cost about $250K. There are people here who have been receiving treatment five times as week for the last three months. There are so many people who simply could not get the treatment they need without a facility like Hope Lodge.

But then, after the initial emotional impact, something else magical happens. You meet other people, and everybody here is lovely. Nobody is down, nobody complains, nobody is mean. And trust me, with the ailments we have, this could be the biggest pity party in town. You may ask about the type of cancer someone has, and you may talk about the cancer for a couple of minutes, but then the conversations run from shopping to current international events. The topics of discussion have incredible range, incredible interest.

Part of the reason is just how the place is run. I also believe that the people here are a special subgroup, in the sense that all of us gave up close proximity to home and the personal support of friends and family in order to receive treatment at a cancer center that meant something special to us. In other words, nobody just ends up here. Every patient here is fighting this disease with a special medical team that was chosen over the sacrifice of leaving home. I feel part of a very special group, a miraculous family.

Alright. I am still quite tired, which is normal, and will continue to be so for a long while. Getting out of bed in the morning takes hours. I usually perk up around noon, crash in the afternoon, perk up again in the afternoon, crash again, and then wake up in the wee hours of the morning, unable to sleep for a couple hours, much to my chagrin. I cannot believe that when I asked why my vision was blurry, I was told the extent of the chemo included changes to the curvatures of the lenses of my eyes! I lost most of my hair, and there is nothing uglier than a light scalp with a sprinkling of black hair. My head looks like a sea cucumber or some other sea creature that lives in the dark. I can easily scare little children. I also lost about twenty pounds. YIPPEE!

$250K for an all-inclusive guaranteed weight-loss program! The only problem is the food sucked, and there were NO FREE MARGARITAS! I had the absolute best care in the hospital (Weill-Cornell a.k.a. Columbia a.k.a. NY Presbyterian Hospital). From the doctors to the housekeeper, everybody was always proactively trying to make things better. I was very lucky. I had minimal mouth sores, no esophageous sores, minimal nausea, limited gastric issues, and limited pain. Except for four days where I don't remember much, I was relatively perky. There were only two out of the twenty days spent in the hospital when I was too exhausted to take a shower. I understand most people suffer more. The day I was discharged, we came to Hope Lodge. I took a nap, and then Wai and I walked half a block to Korea Town, where we proceeded to eat hot spicy Korean Chinese fusion food. It was one of the best meals of my life! My doctor approves yet sighs. I may be the only stem cell transplant patient who celebrated the hospital release with hot chili paste!

I leave Hope Lodge on June 8 and then live at the studio in Manhattan for several weeks. I should know in three to four weeks if the stem cell transplant was successful. I miss the kids so much! Wai has been wonderful. He kept those café lattes coming!

An interesting story to share . . . I was with a new dear friend, Michael, and we took a cab to eat dinner at the 2nd Avenue Deli—which is no longer on Second Avenue. We shared a hot pastrami on rye, ate some potato latkes, downed mustard and half-sour pickles, and then got ready to leave. Michael inquired about their future opening of a second location on the Upper East Side. The manager told him it was going to happen soon. Then he turns around to me and says, "I remember you." To which I answered, "Not in this location." He tells me, "No, no, the old place on Second Avenue, about thirty years ago. You were a student at NYU, studying something brainy, not artsy." Now think carefully—thirty years and thirty pounds ago—AND I DON'T RECOGNIZE MYSELF RIGHT NOW! (Creature from the deep sea, remember?) I look at him astounded; I cannot for the life of me fathom how he could recognize me. He said he remembered me because the first time I went there, I made a fuss about the artificial creamer they served with their coffee, the waitress got mad at me, and he had to sit down and explain what keeping kosher meant.

Once a PITA, always a PITA.

Love,
Olivia

PS: Funny he didn't recognize me with hair when I went there with Mary.

From: Mary Nielsen                       Sent: 06/01/09 7:12 AM
To: "Olivia"
Cc:
Subject: RE: Hope Lodge

Hot chili paste?!?!?!??! Poor Dr. Niesvizky and Dr. Mark! They must be wondering what kind of patient they have. They'll probably win a Nobel Prize for the hot chili paste stem cell cure. What's next after kimchee?!

All is well at your house. We had tacos last night. Plan on chicken tonight. Sounds like you are getting better food than we are. Go figure!

We've been bowling a lot on the Wii. Real smart move, getting that game. It's been keeping us occupied in the evening.

Katie's off to her field trip today to the Lackawanna coalmines. I persuaded her to take an umbrella because it is raining. Hope she doesn't use it down in the mines!

Joe just had a root canal. He's doing fine. I'd be whimpering, but he's back at work already.

Glad all is going well. Say hello to your brother for me. Hope to see you soon.

Mary.

PS: What's a PITA?

Mary,

Thank you taking care of my brood. Two years ago, when you sold your house in Owego and moved in with us for the work week, who knew it was going to be for more than the few weeks to find a new place? And when things got bad last year, it was great to have a third adult to make sure the cherubs got shuttled to and from events. When the stem cell transplant hit, I took it as a divine sign that you were still with us on weekdays. Having you there, knowing my kids' comfort level with "Auntie Mary," has given me something more valuable than any gift. Thank you for providing us with peace of mind.

Gervlyne tells me she has dropped off food a couple of times. Isn't she a fantastic cook? Her Haitian cooking is soooo good. She also is quite familiar with Katie's food intolerances.

I hope Joe is all right. Root canals aren't fun.

It was good to talk to you on the phone. I know things are tough at work right now, but I have had to put things in perspective. Getting laid off at one point of my career would have seemed devastating. Right around now, it would just be another small speed bump on the road of life. What we are more worried about than the loss of income would be the potential loss of benefits. Wai and I have even considered moving to Canada!

To answer your question:

P: Pain
I: In
T: The
A: A*s

Love,
Olivia

Owego Girl Asks Obama Not To Cut VH-71
Ted Fioraliso

June 11, 2009

OWEGO—As we've reported, hundreds of jobs are on the line at Lockheed Martin, after the federal government cut the VH-71 presidential helicopter program.

And one young lady tried to head off the lay-offs by going directly to the top.

"One morning when I was getting up and ready to leave, there was a folded piece of paper, and I'm reading it, and I was quite touched," said Diane Bell of Owego.

That piece of paper was a letter Bell's daughter Hailey asked her to mail. And it was addressed to the President of the United States.

It read, "Dear Mr. President, my name is Hailey Bell and I'm an 11-year-old from Owego, NY. Both my parents work at Lockheed Martin. Lockheed is the main job source in Owego. The presidential helicopter program is a big program. If you shut down the program, my mom may lose her job, and a lot of other people too."

Hailey told President Obama she thinks Owego will become a "ghost town" if he cuts the program.

"It wouldn't be as populated. And we just got voted the Coolest Small Town in America, so that would be kind of sad," said Hailey.

"She's just a very caring person," said Diane. "It didn't surprise me that she wanted to take action."

But that was in April, and since then, the president announced he would cut the program.

Hailey has yet to hear back from the president.

"I know that the president's pretty busy, and I wouldn't expect to get one right away," said Hailey.

Diane says it's OK if they don't get a response—she's just proud of her daughter for stepping up.

"One small thing can have a big effect, and if you're the person who does it, then you're taking action into your own hands," said Hailey.

Although Diane works on the VH-71 project, her husband doesn't. So, she's hopeful their family will weather the storm.[1]

---

[1] Reprinted with permission from and acknowledgment to WENY-TV News

From: Olivia Chin (oliviac@yahoo.com)    Sent: 06/12/09 11:32 AM
To: Friendlist
Cc:
Subject: Sauerkraut and Bottled Water

Hello friends . . .

We left Hope Lodge and moved into the flat that friends we've known
from college are lending us. Thank you, Helene and Dennis! Hope
Lodge was wonderful, nurturing, and luxurious. Because we furnished
the studio with inflatable beds, folding chairs, and folding tables, this is
less comfortable than Hope Lodge. There is much to be said, however,
for a private kitchen, a space filled with windows and light, and a return
to normalcy. Mentally, I am so glad to be here in the studio! A home
away from home . . .

*We broke down and bought two comfy chairs.*

Before leaving Hope Lodge, my brother babysat me. He was in NYC for
a conference, and he finished his week by staying with me and giving Wai
time to get back to Owego to see the girls' dance recital. Did I mention
through all this that Wai managed to attend two dance competitions in
Syracuse as well? Anyway, I was with my brother, Nicky, and we went
to see the doctors on a very rainy day. Now keep in mind I am on this
neutroponic diet. This means no fresh fruit, no fresh veggies, no sushi
or steak tartar, no rare meats, and none of my favorite stinky cheeses.
Not to mention only certain types of bottled water and individually
packaged condiments. I get to the hospital, Dr. Mark asks me, "What's
new?" Nothing much but a touch of nausea, some itchiness. "What have
you been eating?" Mostly Korean food. Then Dr. Niesvizky appears, and
Dr. Mark asks me to tell him about our eating spicy Korean food from
the day we were discharged. Dr. Niesvizky laughs, asks about the nausea,
and then asks what we had last night for dinner, to which I hesitated and
was quickly picked up by Dr. Mark, like a hawk, zoning in for the kill.
"SO WHAT DID YOU EAT LAST NIGHT??" I sheepishly replied,
"Nathan's hot dogs with sauerkraut from the communal bin, mustard
from the communal pump, onion rings, and French fries drowned with
cheese sauce and bacon strips—and ketchup in the little packages! Dr.

Mark looks at me, stunned, and decides this touch of nausea is not a result of chemo.

*I believe nothing grows in mustard or sauerkraut. Have you ever seen anything grow in that jar of mustard that's been in your fridge for the last decade?*

On our way back to Hope Lodge, in the pouring rain, we are about one hundred feet from the door. My brother and I are talking when a cab hits a large puddle and sends a huge wall of street water our way. We are both dripping and drenched to the bone, and I get a mouthful of NYC street puddle water. I spit. We run back to Hope Lodge—and I am not swallowing. My brother races into the room and quickly rips open a duty-free bag and hands me a bottle of single malt whisky he bought from some airport shop as a gift for a friend. I swig. I gargle. My few mouth sores burn. I run to the bathroom, with my brother yelling, "Swallow! Don't spit! It's a two-hundred-dollar bottle of malt whisky!" I spit, brush my teeth, and all I can think about is Lucy screaming, "Germs! ACK! Germs!," after she is kissed by Snoopy. I am worried I will wake up later that night delirious with fever and end up back in the hospital. The next morning, I wake up to find my brother anxiously hovering over me. "How do you feel?" I reply, "I'm hungry."

*So, Dr. Mark, do you think I can stop drinking that bottled water now?*

Strength is coming back in spurts. Wai was here for an entire week again, and we pushed my limits almost every day. While I had stopped taking naps at Hope Lodge, I started again at the studio. My blood counts are also returning to normal ranges, which is fantastic. I haven't had a single transfusion since the discharge from the hospital, and I am told I could be the poster child for stem cell transplants. Humpff! Once my white blood count reached the normal range, Wai and I started venturing farther and longer. We made it to Chinatown one day, and Macy's the next. We started taking buses instead of cabs. Louise, my godmother, came for five days and just left yesterday. She was great company. We went for outings everyday as well. Now I am strong enough to be on my own. My first day on my own, I did laundry, I cleaned, and I slept for over fourteen hours!

Chemotherapy is an interesting thing. It is intended to kill cancer cells without killing too many normal cells, and so the drugs target rapidly dividing tumor cancer cells. The drugs kill the target cells, but they also kill other rapidly dividing cells, such as those in bone marrow, hair follicles, and those in the digestive tract lining. My stem cells repopulated my bone marrow, I am still bald, and I must have a cast-iron digestive system because there were no issues there. I will not know for another two to three weeks whether any of this is working in terms of my M-proteins, kappa-lambda ratios and so on, but I keep praying. The neuropathy in my right foot is actually getting more painful, which is to be expected as the body starts to regenerate neural networks and new synapses start to fire and misfire. However, the really intense ache is gone, and I am pleased to say that I am no longer on mind-numbing painkillers. Just being able to get out of bed, walk around, and get through the day without popping Percocets like candy every three to four hours or so is worth it so far!

*Just my luck—no hair growth yet on my head—but a mustache is sprouting!*

Love,
Olivia

From: WaiCh                                    Sent: 06/18/09 9:04 AM
To: Olivia
Cc:
Subject: Forwarding memo
FYI.
Wai

**From:** Hewson, Marillyn A
**Sent:** Tuesday, June 16, 2009 1:01 PM
**Subject:** Reduction in Force—Self-Nomination

# Memorandum

DATE: June 16, 2009

TO: Lockheed Martin Systems Integration—Owego Employees

FROM: Marillyn Hewson, President

SUBJECT: Reduction in Force—Self-Nomination

As a result of the ongoing workload analysis and critical skills review due to the termination of the VH-71 Presidential Helicopter program, we have determined that approximately 750 positions are at risk for an upcoming reduction in force.

As communicated previously, we have been working to mitigate the impact to jobs. These efforts have included seeking work share within the Corporation, reducing discretionary costs, and identifying employment opportunities within the Corporation for those colleagues affected by our previous reduction in force in May.

Today we are announcing the introduction of a self-nomination option for those employees who wish to leave the business, with entitlement to severance benefits detailed by Corporate policy if selected. Given the magnitude of the reduction in force required, along with direct feedback from employees seeking such a program, it is our hope that the self-nomination option will help reduce the number of employees negatively impacted by the reduction in force. Details on the timeline and self-nomination process are provided in the attached memorandum from Chris Wronsky, vice president of Human Resources. Also attached is the self-nomination form.

Following an assessment of the number of employees who self-nominate, we expect to notify employees affected by the reduction in force around mid-July.

Despite the impact of the termination of the VH-71 program, we are a strong business with a healthy backlog and stable growth plan. Recent announcements we have made this past week on our delivery of the 200th Common Cockpit™ avionics suite for the MH-60R/S multimission helicopter and our selection as an associate prime contractor on the A-10 are indicators of the strength of the business and future growth.

Thank you for your steady focus on performance and customer satisfaction as we work through these changes in our business. I appreciate your dedication and commitment.

From: Cindy Stevens                    Sent: 06/23/2009 1:15 PM
To: "Olivia Chin"
Cc:
Subject: Mambo

Hey There, Girl,

It sounds like you are doing great, I am so happy. We are all fine. My mother is in the hospital this week, a kidney infection—she needs IV antibiotics, Dad's doing fine. Like your kids, mine are finally out of school, and they are ready to burn off energy. I am almost done after this week—nothing for a month YEAH!

Wai called, and Mambo heads home on Sunday. He has really grown on us and fits in like a glove. I'm sure the girls and you miss him, but if you ever need a place for him to stay we'd love to have him. My kids want to keep him! I would steal him in a flash, but you and the girls would go through Mambo withdrawal. He is quite a character! He has gotten used to being with my dogs and running around the house, so I hope he adjusts to being back home. Sorry if he turns out too spoiled! That is the danger of hanging around my home!

Mambo is a wild child. The neighbor called the police last night because Mambo was in the house barking like a maniac. Now this is the neighbor who has called on my dogs before and is a real sour puss, so it is not a concern. But I think Mambo has gotten so used to being with people that when I left him with the other dogs for the night, he decided to raise a little hell. So poor Wai may be in for a shock . . . hee hee.

I am sure you are anxious to get home, but at least you are in your favorite city. Now if it were me, I'd be yelling, "Get me out of here!" A weekend is okay, but that is about it. I would want my own bed and sit in the backyard staring at the birds. Mambo and Dao keep the other critters out. Leave it to you for finding a bead store! I would be in my room, crying in my beer.

I head to St Luke's this weekend to work. I was in Philly last night because I took Tripp to CHOPS. He now has the orthodontic spacer to go next to prepare his gum line for the bone transplant to close the cleft hole that is left. The problem is I was told insurance agencies have a problem with orthodontics, as they see it as cosmetic and not as medically necessary, so I may have a fight on my hands. Oh, well, not the first time.

Keep in touch.

Hugs, Cindy
Mom to Grace, Hope, Faith, and Tripp
"The Best Things in Life Aren't Things"

From: Olivia Chin (oliviac@yahoo.com)    Sent: 06/24/2009 8:48 PM
To: "Nick You"; "Cindy Stevens"
Cc:
Subject: Test Results

Dear Cindy and Nicky,

Funny you two are the only ones interested in test results. Attached are the ones we chose to plot. It goes without saying that we have entered every result in a spreadsheet. The blue and red lines indicate normal min and max ranges.

Once a geek, always a geek.

*Love,*
*Olivia*

WBC

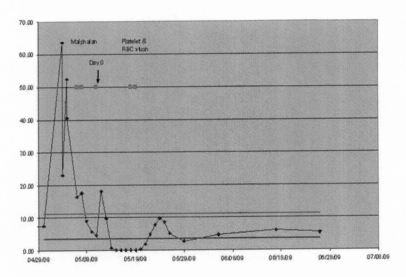

RBC

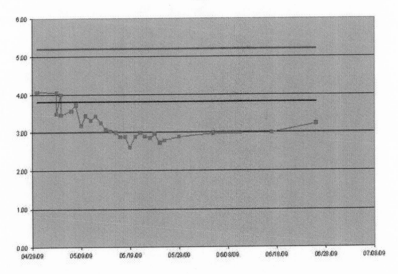

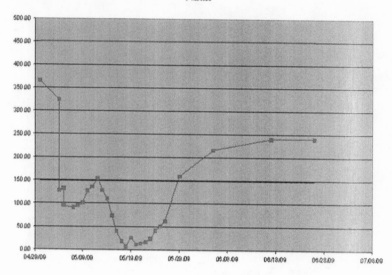

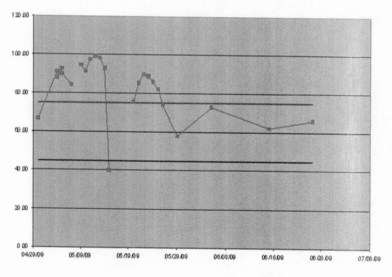

IgG

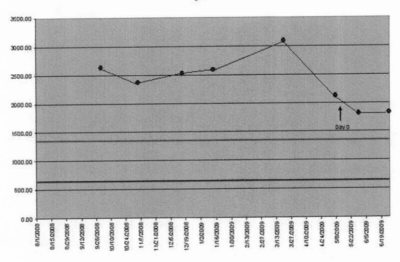

MProtein

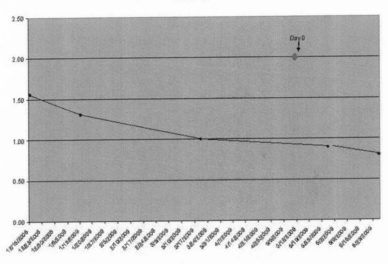

From: Olivia Chin (oliviac@yahoo.com)  Sent: 06/27/09 10:23 AM
To: Friendlist
Cc:
Subject: No More Café Lattes

Dear Friends,

I have been in the Manhattan studio now for several weeks, gaining strength and endurance and learning the hard way not to overdo it. Last week, I met a lovely friend, Eileen, for lunch to celebrate her last day of six weeks of radiation. She was going home! We lunched at a wonderful café about twelve blocks away, and since it was a great day, I decided to walk there. We had a delicious lunch. For dessert, she highly recommended the molten chocolate lava cake. The taste of chocolate is still not what it should be, but the cake was scrumptious. I will simply have to return when my taste buds revive. For whatever reason, instead of taking the bus back as originally planned, I decided to stroll back to the studio. My stroll progressively slowed. By the time I was two blocks away and dragging, I seriously contemplated taking the bus for a single stop! Straggling back, I got to the studio and fell asleep. The next two days, I could hardly move! Everything hurt! So I have learned to read the signs of fatigue, and interestingly enough, the main signal is that my sight goes funky. Everything glares with crazy contrast.

Louise came and left. Her company was a delight. We went out everyday and shopped and ate. Evenings we sat and chatted. I have been on my own now for about two weeks.

Last week was wonderful. Wai surprised me with the girls and dropped by on his way down to the Chesapeake. We hugged and we snuggled, we sat with thighs touching—it had been six weeks since I saw Katie and Elizabeth. They stayed here Thursday night and left for Maryland Friday morning. I should add that they are currently contributing to the pandemonium at Michele and Mike's, who are hosting our girls for two weeks. They have four children of their own. Can you imagine? I am forever indebted to all of you who have taken over the girls—and, in a very selfish way, I am also thrilled that the girls are getting to know all of you better.

I had a medical appointment on Friday. Wai woke us all up early, and we went to Chinatown for breakfast at 7:30! Katie had a honeydew slushee. We all had congee and rice flour crepes with shrimp. Yum! Then we headed uptown to Cornell Medical, where we found a lovely place to sit and hang out for the short wait before my early appointment. Wai and the girls were getting ready to leave. Katie gave me a great big hug and whispered sweet good-byes. Elizabeth, who has difficulty saying good-bye, gave me a quick hug. Then she returned to give me a huge hug and started crying and sobbing while clasping me around my neck. All of a sudden, Elizabeth stopped in mid-hiccup, and I heard Katie say those words a mother never wants to hear: "Uh oh."

Elizabeth had sprouted a bloody nose. And we were not dealing with the garden variety of bloody noses. We were dealing with the Red Sea. As Katie wiped my back off with tissues, Elizabeth continued to gush like a small fountain. Surrounded by soaked red tissues, Katie had the delicate touch to comment that it was a bloody good thing we were in a hospital. After the flow was staunched, Elizabeth tried to give me another good-bye hug. We all parted laughing, as I made signs to ward her off as if she was a vampire, and she tried to advance toward me.

Then I saw Dr. Mark. Although still too early to make any assessment, he had the results of the blood test with one of the significant markers. The marker is the M-protein, which was 0.1 lower than the previous reading. Although not yet significant, I interpret this as a positive sign. At least it did not increase!

With this last visit, the morning delivery of café lattes ceased. Wai had been spoiling me. When confronted, he simply said, "The ninety-nine-cent special is over." Sigh. I am apparently not worth more than ninety-nine cents.

Otherwise, life is simple. Fill what's empty, empty what's full, scratch where it itches. Since we splurged for high-speed and wireless Internet and scrimped on cable, there is not much to watch. There are infomercial channels, Latino channels, Chinese channels, a 24/7 panning of major NYC traffic intersections, and the local network channels. So guess what I watch? You got it! The Food Network.

I have been told by everyone from volunteers, nurses, social workers, and physicians that I have been exceptionally lucky with my stem cell transplant. Minimal nausea, minimal mouth sores, and just a few days of gastric distress, and enough energy on most days to shower, read, bead, and feed. Upon discharge, the lucky streak continued, with my ability to eat kimchee and spicy Korean food for the first two weeks, followed by just about anything but the kitchen sink. My doctors think I have a cast iron stomach. The luck continues with the level of fatigue, which I think is high, but I am assured is exceptionally low. I have been fortunate enough since the transplant to only have one single responsibility: to get better. This is being done with a lot help from friends and much effort from Wai. I am not home, where I would have the words *mother, wife,* and *dog walker* emblazoned upon me, probably in huge scarlet letters. I am not home, where my beloved family would look at me every day at six p.m. and bellow "What's for dinner?" I am not home to deal with dust, mildew, plants, dog, and kids. Sometimes I miss my family so much, it hurts. Then the thought of lugging groceries home and cooking for a family who feeds like raptors hits, and I sigh. I sure miss those ravenous raptors!

Love,
Olivia


PS: I gained back eight pounds. I wonder how that happened?

From: Olivia Chin (oliviac@yahoo.com) Sent: 07/01/09 9:37 PM
To: Michele
Cc:
Subject: Hostages

Hi, Michele!

I figure you are not answering your cell phone for one of the following reasons:

1) The kids are so noisy, you wouldn't be able to hear a fire engine siren, let alone your cell phone ringtone.
2) You are tied up to a chair, there is a streak of hair missing through the top of your head where the kids shaved you, and you have masking tape over your mouth.
3) The kids got your cell phone and dropped it into the Chesapeake.
4) You are so tired from watching six kids, you are nodding off throughout the day, and you turned off your cell phone in order to nap.
5) The kids are at the bottom of the Chesapeake along with your cell phone, and you are in Bora Bora.
6) You have spent the day waiting at triage at the ER.
7) You are driving to Owego and bringing my girls back home early.
8) Mike is driving all six kids to Owego for Wai to watch them.
9) You have no time at all to yourself; by the time the zoo has been fed and the kitchen is cleaned up, it's already time for the next feeding.
10) The kids are tied to chairs, they have no hair left on their heads, and they have masking tape over their mouths. If you answer the phone, the stony background silence is a dead giveaway for anyone on the other end of the phone to call 911.

Love you. Thank you. Wai is finally going to be able to get to the house, the lawn, the bills, the insurance . . . and possibly get to work. I don't even ask him about the pool, which according to my kids looks like the spawning ground for the creature of the green lagoon.

Love,
Olivia

From: Olivia Chin (oliviac@yahoo.com)  Sent: 07/02/2009 11:31AM
To: "Nick You"
Cc:
Subject: Post-Treatment Blues

Dear Nicky,

Just some random and rambling thoughts today. For over twenty days, I was in the hospital, with a very structured schedule. Except for a few emergencies involving neighboring patients, I was largely unaware of the outside world. By that, I mean anything outside the double doors to my room. And so anybody who came into the room was there for me. I was poked, prodded, pricked, and applauded. I was the focus of anyone who came near me. Even Wai spoiled me; he has never been so attentive.

Then came Hope Lodge and now the studio. I think I was too tired at Hope Lodge to notice the first signs of grey that crept in toward the end of my stay there. Then the grey hit.

I am here alone; the appointments with Dr. Mark and Dr. Niesvizky are getting spaced further and further apart. Wai calls me once or twice a day to make sure I am alive. The treatment over, the daily routine over, now the waiting game begins. I do not know if the treatment had the desired effect of putting this disease in remission. So here I sit, with this body that has betrayed me once already, waiting, in the game of life.

I asked Dr. Mark, what if? He tells me if this procedure was not successful, we'll go for Stem Cell Transplant Number Two. Just what I wanted to hear. A second transplant may very well be in the future anyway because remission is not forever. I am hoping it is in the distant future. He gave a wonderful presentation on a relatively new drug therapy; it shows promise of prolonged remission. He says I will be able to start this new treatment on Day 100. I was so depressed after the presentation as the reality of this situation returned. I want this disease to be gone forever. I want a younger, more nubile, healthy body! I want . . . I want . . .

I want to live to what should be my normal life expectancy.

Love,
Olivia

From: EileenE Sent: 07/04/2009 1:47 PM
To: "Olivia Chin"
Cc:
Subject: Post-Treatment Blues

Dear Olivia,

Your thoughts mirror those in the article I've recently read in the *New York Times*, "Losing a Comforting Ritual: Treatment" by Dana Jennings. In it, he writes about the unexpected post-treatment letdown. He compares the post-treatment period to getting fired or laid off.

I guess these feelings are very common and not discussed often enough, probably because the doctors are only concerned with healing us, not with our psyches. That's our problem. I wonder if support group facilitators have ever discussed this or are even aware that cancer patients have these feelings. I will be attending a lung cancer support group very soon, and I will bring it up and see how much awareness there is about this very real problem.

Meanwhile, it's comforting to know that we're not alone with this, and just knowing that is very helpful. One less black thought to cope with.

Cyberhug,
Eileen

From: Olivia Chin (oliviac@yahoo.com)  Sent: 07/07/09 8:17 AM
To: Friendlist
Cc:
Subject: Read, Bead, and Feed

Dear Friends,

I had a brief bout with post-treatment letdown, a term referred to and possibly coined by Dana Jennings at the *NY Times* in a recent article about his treatment. It was a relief to know that others share similar sensations. Feeling disconnected to everything, I was decidedly in a fog of a funk. It crept up when I wasn't looking. Then one night, as I was watching nothing on television, scooping out the insides of a large honeydew with a spoon and feeling very sorry for myself, it hit me that I had to get out of the grey. It was decidedly a very bad and unflattering shade of grey.

So I went to a bookstore and bought some fun fantasy reading for young adults. I disappeared into a world populated by fairies and elves for a couple of days.

I found a beautifully landscaped public terrace on top of a tall building with benches, tables, and pergolas. Then the wet weather of the last month stopped, and we had some glorious sunny days. Guess where I was enjoying the sun?

I went to lunch in Chinatown. Then I went shopping there and bought some huge scallops. I cooked them and ate these delicious morsels for dinner. It took two days to get the fishy smell out of the studio.

Then Louise and Sal dropped by with gifts of food. They took me out to lunch at a diner. The food was very good, and the company even better.

I beaded and made a beautiful pearl necklace. (So modest).

Then Helene and Dennis dropped by. They took me out to dinner at a superb Greek restaurant in Astoria. (Remember the lusty cravings for slices of semolina bread topped with tamaroasalata?) Helene admired the necklace; it's hers now. I went online last night to order more pearls. Shopping is such an uplifting experience!

I feel so much better now.

I saw Dr. Mark today. Did I ever mention that Dr. Niesvizky and Dr. Mark are also foodies? I believe one is a gourmand, the other a gourmet. Or they are both gourmets, and one is also a gourmand. Or they are both, both. Anyway, once I brought them dumplings. Another time, they got black bean paste Chinese cakes. This time, I went to the Magnolia Bakery and bought cupcakes. (This is the only way I know how to show my appreciation to these two men who are saving my life). While at the bakery, I sampled lemon, red velvet, and vanilla cupcakes. They were all delicious! Then I was off to the hospital where they take vitals. I gained eight pounds out of the twenty I lost in the hospital. Now how do you suppose that happened?

There wasn't much to the check-up today, other than some of the answers from Dr. Mark to questions I had caught me by surprise. I didn't know I was supposed to stay out of the sun. (So much for the afternoon sunbaths on that terrace). I didn't know the chemo medication is still in me. (It explains weird side effects that are still current). I didn't know I wasn't supposed to take buses or subways yet. (We've been taking buses for almost a month!) The only reason I haven't taken a subway yet is because it's too hard to go up and down the stairs. Dr. Mark heaved a sigh and acquiesced on the NYC transit buses. I can't swim for another six months. (There is a beautiful pool in the sports club in this building. I packed my swimsuit away). I can only drink a tiny bit of wine at a time. (I decided it was best to avoid asking about his definitions of tiny and the exact periodicity of "at a time." Doesn't that mean small sips very slowly?). Finally, I understood the importance of counting the days from Day Zero, which is the day the stem cells are returned to your body. I am at Day 58. Day 100 is when your body is significantly healed and there is little chemo left in you, so you can take other medications and resume more normal activities.

Every time you go to the Multiple Myeloma Clinic to see a physician, they draw blood for tests. This time, the tests include checking for a significant marker. It takes a week to get the results. So, the seemingly endless wait continues, the healing progresses, and the new routine becomes just the routine.

*Love,*
*Olivia*

PS: My informal survey of tens of thousands of sandal-shod women revealed I was the last woman in this city to have unpainted toenails. So I bought a bottle of nail polish and proceeded to paint my toes and toenails. How does one get nail polish off of one's toes?

From: Olivia Chin (oliviac@yahoo.com)   Sent: 07/13/2009 10:57 AM
To: "Nick You"
Cc:
Subject: Trust

Dear Nicky,

Just sharing some thoughts that have been filtering through my mind recently.

I went to a seminar given by Dr. Mark on a drug therapy for multiple myeloma patients that has shown promise to extend the remission period following chemo or stem cell transplants. This drug is still undergoing clinical trials right now. While there, a patient of another doctor appeared upset to hear about this relatively new drug. He was concerned that he was not on this new drug. Dr. Mark had to explain to him that the chemo drug he was on is the current medical standard. How odd—this man is a patient of Dr. Niesvizky—why wouldn't he trust his doctor? If I did not trust Dr. Mark and Dr. Niesvizky with my life, I would not be seeing them.

Then, after the discussion, another woman approached Dr. Mark. I was waiting to talk to Dr. Mark, but moved away after overhearing her opening remarks to him. She wanted to switch over to be his patient. Once again, it struck me as odd. Why did both of these people distrust their own doctors? Why would they want to switch physicians or medications so quickly?

Last Wednesday, I saw Dr. Mark. While I was there, I went to say hello to Inja, the stem cell collection nurse. This woman is an angel. While there, Inja cleaned the tunneled catheter of a woman. This woman was so upset about this cleaning, claiming it had never been done before. Then when Inja cleaned both tubes, the woman was concerned that she only usually gets one tube cleaned. She started questioning everything that had been done in the past, damning her previous nurses and her physician. As it turns out, the catheter had been cleaned properly before. She got the chemo and cleaning procedures confused. I chalked up her confusion and attitude to ignorance.

Last Friday, I went back to Hope Lodge NYC to have lunch with someone—I dub her X. This is not someone whose company I particularly enjoy. However, I was asked by Eileen to contact her and see how she was doing. Three weeks ago, Eileen knew that this person was supposed to start a new treatment.

I got to Hope Lodge. X had forgotten about our lunch appointment and was still asleep at half past noon. So I waited for over an hour until X was ready to go. We spent almost three hours together—during the entire time, there was not one single positive comment made about anything or anybody except the food. X was still harping about things that had happened well over ten years ago. Then we finally got to her most current problem. X was not responding to her current treatment anymore, and her physician wanted her to switch to a more aggressive chemo. X was not sure this was the right treatment for her. High on her list of concerns is the loss of her hair. Now it turns out her physician is one of the best in this country for her particular cancer—well renowned, well respected, and well published. X has been in stage four cancer for over seventeen years, and this physician is credited for keeping her alive with a high quality of life.

Why is it that none of these people trust their physicians? Do they know more? Are they better versed to make medical decisions than their doctors? I believe in getting second opinions and making informed decisions. I ask a lot of questions, I read information from trusted sources on the Internet. But ultimately, I have to find a physician I trust and pray that he or she makes the best decision possible for me.

*Love,*
*Olivia*

From: Nick You     Sent: 07/16/2009 5:22 PM
To: "Olivia Chin"
Cc:
Subject: RE: Layoffs

Hey, I just did a quick look on the Internet about your area. I found an article in your local paper titled "Lockheed cuts 600 workers: Owego plant sees 25% loss of employees in 2009." It was written by John Hill. What is going on?

Nicky

From: Olivia Chin (oliviac@yahoo.com) Sent: 07/16/2009 6:25 PM
To: "Nick You"
Cc:
Subject: Work

Dear Nicky,

I just thought you would want to know that Wai is still gainfully employed.
When everyone else was sitting at work feeling like one of those ducks in
a row you shoot at in a carnival, Wai was weeding the yard with the girls.
He took the week off. He is planning to take them to a water park later
this week. The kids are bemoaning the fact that he only does one ride
plus the wave pool and the lazy river. They say they wish I were there so
we could scream while hurtling down those black tubes or collide in the
giant vortex ride. I always look at the vortex as the giant version of the
spittoon at the dentists. The one at the dentist is probably cleaner.

I was probably more worried than he. Although I would like to spend
my remaining good years with him at home, we would have had a gap
in health insurance until he was eligible for retirement benefits. Given
my current condition, that is just not an option we can even consider. I
feel like a burden, and it bothers me.

Our area will be devastated. Between the previous recent layoff, the one
today, which impacted about another six hundred people, plus those who
quit and the others who volunteered to take advantage of the incentive
package, about one thousand people have lost their jobs. This represents
about one-fourth of the workforce where Wai works. Since there is no
other large employer in the area, the impact is huge.

A friend, Diane, called this morning to tell me she was laid off. Then she
added, "There are worse things than being laid off. I could be you!" I am
so glad I was able to provide her with some perspective!

Love,
Olivia

From: Olivia Chin (oliviac@yahoo.com)  Sent: 07/23/09 7:21 PM
To: Friendlist
Cc:
Subject: It Takes a Village

Dear Friends,

I go for walks everyday to try to build up strength and muscle tone. It
is also part of the Olivia Financial Stimulus Package. The outings have
ranged from short strolls to the supermarket to longer treks to bead shops.
I even made it to IKEA one day on their free water taxi shuttle just for
fun. The cooler weather earlier this summer has ceased. Hot and humid
here in Manhattan, I am still making my daily outings, but they are no
longer getting more extended each day. It's just too muggy! In addition,
there is now usually one stop somewhere for a large iced tea. I feel like a
true city girl now—I can bellow with the best: "A venti iced half-green
half-black with two syrup shots!"

*Is there such a thing as a tea barista?*

The kids returned from two glorious weeks in Maryland, where they
stayed with Michele and Mike and their four kids in the Chesapeake area.
They then went with a friend, Carol, up on Skaneateles Lake, NY. They
are now in Queens, NY, with Rey and Lisette. They then go on to Helene
and Dennis's on Long Island, before returning to Owego to spend time
with my brother, who is flying in from Kenya next week. They are having
a great time. One of the wonderful outcomes of this blasted disease is that
Katie and Elizabeth and our friends and family are getting to really know
each other. When we visit, typically the adults gather and gab, whilst the
kids play amongst themselves. Now, my friends and family are interacting
directly with the girls. Mambo has been staying off and on with Cindy
Ellen, playing with her dog pack and her four kids. Starting earlier this
year with dance competitions through the end of this summer, I realize
now that a stem cell transplant isn't anything one does alone or even
with a single caregiver. It involves caregivers as well as supporters to the
immediate family. It involves well-wishers and prayers. It involves phone
calls, lodging, food, and cards. The amount of care and support requires
a village. You all are my village. Thank you from the heart.

*Hmm . . . Let's just hope my friends and family don't share too much about my—ahem—model youth with them.*

A luncheon cruise was hosted last weekend by the hospital for stem cell transplant survivors. I was not originally invited—too recent a transplant to be considered—but received an invitation when I asked if I could attend. Technically, I crashed the cruise with Michael. This was held on a charter yacht, and it was lovely. It was so special seeing nurses, administrators, doctors, and social workers again, out of context, out of scrubs. It also struck me how one could not tell the survivors from their guests.

*They must have better wigs than me.*

This week, I went for another medical follow up. I saw Dr. Niesvizky rather than Dr. Mark. I wanted to pick his brain on a clinical trial he is running for a remission chemo drug therapy that is being considered for me. However, since the trial is still ongoing, Dr. Niesvizky chose not to share any data. Drat these doctors with such integrity! The first thing done at the clinic is the recording of vitals. The scale informed me I had gained another two pounds, which resulted in a rather loud profanity from my part. Dr. Niesvizky peered at me and asked what the issue was. I replied that I had gained two more pounds, and I didn't understand why. He smiled and said he had some pretty valid theories about it. Oh, the smugness . . . If I didn't worship the ground he walks on, I would have slugged him. Perhaps I forgot to mention that NYC Restaurant Week is going on for several weeks this month and indulgence in a few too many three-course lunches might be supporting data for his theories? The list of questions was shorter than usual—only fifteen this visit. Toward the end of the visit, I asked Dr. Niesvizky why the few hairs on my head are continuing to fall out while I am sprouting a mustache on just the sides of my mouth. He said they programmed the stem cell transplant program so all the patients end up looking like him!

*Due to ethnic differences, I fear I am slowly morphing into a bald Asian sage with a wispy, long beard.*

I got good news! One of the major markers for response to treatment or disease progression for myeloma is the M-protein. This marker has not been relevant until now due to its thirty-day half-life. (Pass the milk please, Madame Curie). Enough time has finally elapsed so that this marker can start to show if the stem cell transplant had any impact. This marker can be seen through electrophoresis. Electrophoresis is a bit similar to spectrum analysis. It is a method of separating proteins based on their properties while zapping them with electricity. With some other processes, this marker is viewed as a graph with spikes indicating various protein subsets on the x-axis and an indication of quantity on the y-axis. With myeloma, this test usually results in a large spike—too much of a single type. While my M-protein had been declining slowly before, it stayed the same this time at 0.8 g/dl as the sample from about a month ago. I was rather bummed. Then Dr. Niesvizky said there was a second spike at 0.05. I had no idea what this meant. I think he explained to me that this is an indication that the stem cells are starting to produce another form of protein. Around this time, I was taking notes furiously and trying really hard to follow him. I think he said this means my body is now working to eliminate some of the malignant protein clones. He called this an "atypical monoclonal pattern." Then I started poking around papers published by Dr. Niesvizky and Dr. Mark and found a recent one on the subject of atypical serum immunofixation patterns (ASIPs).

*Where do they come up with these acronyms? MGUS, ASIPs—no imagination whatsoever. Don't they know who they are dealing with? Here stands the originator of the Ship Helo Integration and Test Simulator and the Radar Automated Testing System.*

Did you ever take a course where you struggled to follow everything during a seminar and felt you really had a good grasp of it all—only to realize a few hours later that you no longer had any idea what was discussed? I returned to the studio really confused. I searched and read the Internet and got even more confused. I have a call into Dr. Mark to get a better grasp of it all. But the bottom line is the marker shows I am responding to the stem cell transplant well.

*Good. As lovely as everyone was at the hospital, I really don't want to see them again for a second transplant any time soon.*

So I celebrated by going out to eat with Michael.

*Did you expect anything less?*

*Love,*
*Olivia*

PS: Thank you all for your most helpful and most peculiar tips on the recent issue of getting rid of excess toenail polish. First prize is awarded to the originator of "Have Sven lick it off."

From: Olivia Chin (oliviac@yahoo.com)    Sent: 07/27/2009 12:18 PM
To: "Nick You"
Cc:
Subject: Marriage

Dear Nicky,

Since you are breaking up with Wife Number Three and moving on, please allow me to give you some advice.

When Wai and I were dating, we essentially had just started working, so while we had some assets as individuals, we had not yet accumulated a lifetime of stuff. At the time, a prenuptial agreement seemed a farce as well as a premonition of marital doom.

Today, I think differently. I just spoke to a friend, whose wife had cancer. Her treatment resulted in major brain damage. She is a changed person. He is the caregiver and husband to a woman he no longer loves. He is still in love with the woman he married. I have another friend who wiped out on a boogie board in Chile and is wheelchair-bound due to spinal injuries. Another colleague fell from a small hill during an introductory hang gliding lesson and is disabled physically and mentally. This afternoon, I am going to provide moral support to Eileen, a friend who has lung cancer. She is hearing for the first time the results of her scan last week, taken with enough elapsed time to provide insight as to the effectiveness of her six weeks of radiation.

Incurable terminal diseases and accidents—they happen. The Really Bad Stuff does hit. I have boiled down this sorry soup into three parts: this damn disease, love, and money.

This Damn Disease:
I told Wai he had my permission to check me into a nursing home when the time comes. I also told him that I may not be of sound mind by then, and if I do not agree, he can hold me to my agreement now and ignore any protests in the future. It is not being unselfish—it's the issue of this damn disease. *Why should it ruin both of our lives?* As it is, it is consuming a large chunk of our lives. Wai said that when the bad times hit, he hopes

he will be retired and can spend time taking care of me. I told him he is not going to spend his retirement wiping my bloomin' arse! On the flip side, I know I would hesitate checking him into a facility. I suppose if the outlook was short, caring for a loved one might be the best way to deal with saying good-bye. If the outlook were very extended, I would want him to be free.

Love:
When we got married, I told Wai I did not believe in divorce. Murder maybe, but not divorce. Then, when we had bad fights, I would dig these really deep trenches in the backyard. Usually after a trench was dug, he would behave really well for quite awhile. When the back and foot pain got so bad last year I was no longer able to dig, four girlfriends signed up for the Secret Digging Committee. It really ticks me off that I can no longer run him over in the driveway. I need the medical benefits. *It's not fun depending on anyone.* Of course, I want someone who loves me to take care of me. But I would rather see Wai's smiling face once every few days with a big café latte in hand than to see him turn into a grumpy old man. It's called love. I love him with all my heart. And this is a crappy thing that happened to me. And it is a crappy thing that is happening to him. I love him enough that I do not want to drag him down with me.

Money:
There may be certain advantages to being divorced. I have been mulling them over. The question boils down to whether one gets divorced out of love or to gain insurance coverage. One is done with honor, the latter is system abuse. With the recent layoffs in our area, I have wondered if we would be better off with my being on my own and on disability. I found out during this process that I do still love Wai very much. But I also found out I am not afraid of living alone. I would prefer not to live without him, but I can. And in the end, if it benefits everyone, it is a choice to be considered. Am I going to burn through the funds we set aside for the girls' college? Should I spend everything we put aside for the both of us? Will the medical and care expenses eat up all we have worked for? This is an interesting time for us to be considering the potential health care reform.

Anyway, if you should embark on another relationship with any sort of commitment, my advice to you is to discuss how you want to handle not only the dissolution of the relationship, but to also discuss how you expect to handle The Really Bad Stuff. After all, you are almost eight years older than me. A spring chicken you are no longer, and you may be nearing The Really Bad Stuff earlier than me! (How's that for a really compassionate touch?)

Last—I need to add that Lockheed Martin has the most amazing benefits. Did you know that there are two nurses indirectly paid from Lockheed assigned to keeping in touch with me and making sure everything is getting taken care of with a minimum of hassle? One is a general nurse, and one handles stem cell transplants. Between the two of them, I can usually expect a call every two weeks. They have answered many questions, and they even have taken care of insurance problems we have encountered. Amazing.

*Love and Clucks,*
*Olivia*

From: Olivia Chin (oliviac@yahoo.com)   Sent: 08/12/09 7:42 PM
To: Friendlist
Cc:
Subject: I really need to update my MP3 (still in the Age of Aquarius)

Dear Friends,

There are extended periods when I see nobody. Then I see so many
people it makes my head spin! Two weeks ago, Gervlyne stopped by
to see me—I was so happy to see her! Whenever we are together, we
laugh and laugh. My other laughing best bud from college is Toan
who now lives in Vietnam; he came to visit with his ten-year-old son,
Matthew, the same weekend as Gervlyne. I never knew Toan when
he was a young kid, but Matthew provided us with a glimpse of what
once was. Helene and Dennis came into town with Katie and Elizabeth.
Helene picked the girls up from Rey and Lisette's. Then Wai came. Toan,
Helene, and I used to hang out in college. It has been twenty-seven
years since the three of us had been together! It took this damn disease
to reunite us. The highlight of the trip was introducing Matthew to
cannolis at Veniero's Café and Bakery. As students, Toan and I used to
live four blocks away from Veniero's. We would buy treats there to go,
eating them right out of the box, too cheap to pay for cappuccinos, café
lattes, and tips. We brought Matthew there Friday night. It was love at
first bite. Saturday, after dinner, Matthew begged us on his knees to go
back for more cannolis. Little did he know that we did not need much
incentive. Matthew left gratified and grinning, clutching two more mini
cannolis, destined for his breakfast.

*Reunited, and it feels so good!*

One of the most startling things about this city is how much it has
changed. About thirty years ago, the eastside neighborhood known as
Alphabet Soup was at best a hostile environment. Hell's Kitchen was
hell. The west side was the Wild, Wild West. I used to walk back to
my apartment with my keys splayed between my fist fingers. Ladies
of the night beckoned from doorways, along with drug pushers,
pimps, and junkies. There were homeless people, living in cardboard
shantytowns—one even sported a teepee. Now, it seems there are

no really bad or scary neighborhoods in Manhattan anymore. I have not ventured all over, but the streets are cleaner, buildings have been scrubbed, and there are potted plants and flowering hanging baskets along major thoroughfares. Alphabet Soup is trendy, Hell's Kitchen, even more so. I am also amazed at the many accommodations for the handicapped. I ♥ NY!

*I'm in a New York state of mind . . .*

Then Edith, a friend we met in China when we were adopting Elizabeth, came to visit. Helene and I met several times and took advantage of Restaurant Week, which is now going into its second month! We had Chinese and Greek lunch specials, in case you were wondering. Add to that a few more fabulous lunches with Michael, including one at Le Cirque (just to be able to cattily drop a name). I had two appointments with Dr. Mark. (Am I here for medical reasons or to eat my way through NYC?) The first visit necessitated another trip to Veniero's for treats for his staff. And breakfast for me. Then I went on a trip to DC to attend an informative two-day seminar by the International Myeloma Foundation. Exhausting. After that trip, I was so tired I didn't even want to get out of PJs, and reverted to taking daily naps. So a little incentive was sorely needed to get out of the studio. I headed down to Jacques Torres, chocolate maker, for a frozen Wicked Chocolate—icy and spicy! And tried a sample of their goods. I then had to compare it to the quayaquil at La Maison du Chocolat. I am trying to walk it all off. At the rate of current consumption, I need to walk to Owego and back in the next week. In case you are wondering, the scale at the doctors' office has not ejected any springs or flashed error codes in protest yet.

*He ain't heavy, he's my brother.*

Dr. Mark had to reclarify that which had been explained so well by Dr. Niesvizky, which was then distorted by this mind of mine. It is amazing the mind games that are played when one is anxiously anticipating results of significant tests. Dr. Mark was able to confirm that I am responding well to the stem cell transplant. They have detected two bands of my M-protein. The presence of two M-proteins indicates that I'm an ASIP (atypical serum immunofixation pattern), which is good news. I also had a MRI done due to pain between the shoulder blades. Once again, while waiting for the medical test results, my mind decided to follow every dark recess, chase every deadly doubt. Early this year, I had a PET-CT scan in which vertebrae T4 glowed, indicating increased cancerous activity. I convinced myself I had lesions in my spine and that T4 was just a thing of the past. This MRI showed a spine with little or no myeloma activity, with some arthritis present. That was also good news. I think I cured myself of the "waiting for results" game after this last session of "reality—what a concept!" I've decided to stop waiting for results and tests and doctors' visits and to start living life instead. I am living with myeloma; I am not dying of it.

*Oh, girls, they wanna have fu-un . . .*

After seeing Dr. Mark (and saying hello to Dr. Niesvizky), Inja (the angel nurse) took me back to the stem cell transplant unit to talk to a patient. It was odd going back to that ward. She was at day five of her transplant. I was at day eight-one. It gave this patient a boost to know that eventually the fatigue fades, the nausea lessens, and life resumes. Then I came back to the studio to find my second order of beads had arrived! A three-pound box of beads—it doesn't take much to make me happy! I've developed a new line of charm bracelets, the proceeds of which will be going to The Joseph Michaeli Fund for myeloma research. The bracelet themes are: cooking mama, party mama, vino mama, beach mama, and weeding mama. (The latter includes gardening-themed charms, not cannabis you wicked, wicked friends of mine!) Some of these are currently in the display case at the NYU Cancer Clinic boutique. Front and Center in Owego will soon be sporting "cooking mama" bracelets! I am going to try Sloan Kettering next.

*Lucy in the sky with diamonds . . .*

I go home at the end of August. I will miss this city, which has helped heal me, but I need to go home to be with my family. Mambo is going to get a lot of exercise—I am determined to keep up the daily walks. Another sign from the divine: I had my head shaved, and a week later, little stubs started growing. No longer do I sport the sea cucumber look. Everyone, check out the baby cactus on my head!

*Gimme a head with hair, long, beautiful hair*

Love,
Olivia

From: Olivia Chin (oliviac@yahoo.com)       Sent: 08/19/09 3:07 PM
To: Friendlist
Cc:
Subject: Fish Rapidly Disappearing from Atlantic

Dear Friends,

It's Day 100!!!

The day one receives the infusion of stem cells is considered Day Zero.
That date for me was May 11, 2009. The following days are referred to
by positive sequential numbers. So Day One would have been May 12.
If you remember, I had the high-dose chemo on Day Minus Four. Day
100 is a significant date because your body is considered significantly
healed and there is so little chemo left in you that so you can take
other medications and resume more normal activities. (I'm not so sure I
waited). Still no crowds—what a bummer! Yo Yo Ma is playing at Lincoln
Center at Mostly Mozart. Sigh. And I missed the entire ballet season here.
BUT . . . BUT . . .

# I CAN HAVE SUSHI !

I called Dr. Mark yesterday, and Patty (one fantastic and extremely capable
assistant) called me back at 5:24 p.m. to say that I could embark on my
efforts to deplete the Atlantic of fish. So guess who was gulping down
raw fish within hours last night on Day 99.5? Forget sushi—I was doing
major damage on sashimi. I would eat sushi in a box. With a fox. I would
eat sushi here and there. I would eat sushi anywhere. However, I am
going to wait on green eggs, even though there is nothing as good as
congee with thousand-year-old eggs. (Should I ask Dr. Mark next week
about green eggs? Or stinky tofu? Or Gorgonzola? Ooh—how about
homemade fermented sticky rice ?)

Lynette and her daughter Paris were in town yesterday for a passport
renewal. It was so good to see them! Lynette reminded me that her
second request to host my kids was denied. Their summer schedules are
full. Next week they are with Judith and Ken. Then I am home! Lynette
gave me two dozen long-stemmed roses in the most cheerful, bright

pink. Had I not been so close to Day 100, these would not have been possible for me to keep. So here I sit on my folding chair, using a laptop on a folding table next to my deflatable bed with two-dozen roses on my collapsible shelves, basking in the glory of Day 100 with the AC going in full arctic-blast mode. (It's hot and muggy outside, detestable weather). I have a mug of fabulous coffee from Zabars beside me. Life is good. So here goes a little something Inja shared with me on Day Minus Five that has helped me so much:

"Do not be anxious about anything, but in everything, by prayer and petition, with thanksgiving, present your requests to God. And the peace of God, which transcends all understanding, will guard your hearts and your minds" (Philippians 4:5-7).

So, dear Supreme Being, a.k.a. Buddha, Jesus, Holy Spirit, God, Elohim, Yahweh, Allah, Adonai, Bhagwan, Krishna, Waheguru, Shen, Odin, Ishwar, and any form you deign to take, be it an eagle flying overhead or the replenished supply of fish in waters that run deep, thank you for the food I take, thank you for the love you make, thank you for the joy you create, help me adjust to life at home, and please, please find a cure for myeloma sometime soon.

Love,
Olivia

Dear Nicky,

It sure was interesting meeting P★★★★a. All I can say is, she appears to be nice. I've decided the criteria of Three Bs in judging your girlfriends needs to be amended. She isn't particularly beautiful, she has some manners, and she is definitely not brainy. What you see in her, I don't know, but I think another B needs to be added to the list:

Beauty, Brains, and Breeding OR male ego-Boosting

I never said I was nice. I'll sign up for beauty, brains, and breeding. God only knows, any man who hangs around me had better be very secure and have the ability to respond with whiplash speed. Or in Wai's case, he ignores me and doesn't respond at all. I think it is his method of self-preservation. Years ago, early in our marriage, we were together in the family room, and he was inspired by some asinine TV show he was watching. In a moment of sheer stupidity, he bellowed at me, "Woman! Bring me a Coke on ice!" He later confessed that he had serious misgivings when he saw me quietly get up and leave for the kitchen. He had some concerns right then about his life expectancy. I came back with a saucer, upon which there was an ice cube dusted with flour, and dumped the saucer and its contents on his lap. I vaguely remember saying something about his having to sleep sometime.

So if P★★★★a makes you happy, and she does not threaten you on a regular basis, we'll stop pecking. Just make sure please that you know why she makes you happy and that the reason is a sound one that can endure.

When I said she was not the sharpest crayon in the box, you looked confused. So here are some fun colloquiums to add to your repertoire.

And thank you for taking care of the girls. They will never forget their time with you.

Love and pecks,
Olivia

### The Sharpest Crayon in the Box

*He's not the sharpest crayon in the box.*
*He's not the brightest light on the tree.*
*She's not the sharpest pencil in the box.*

*She's as sharp as a beach ball.*
*He's got the IQ of a head of cabbage.*
*There's a hollow echo in his hall.*

*The wheel may be turning, but the hamster is dead.*
*She couldn't find her way out of a paper bag.*
*She's not the sharpest tool in the shed.*

*She's not playing with a full deck.*
*He doesn't have both oars in the water.*
*He's a few cards short of a card deck.*

*There are no lights on in the attic.*
*He's a few fries short of a Happy Meal.*
*The TV is on, but there's nothing but static.*

She's dumber than a box of bricks.
He fell off the turnip truck.
She's no rocket scientist.

She's not the sharpest knife in the block.
He's a candidate for the Darwin Award.
He threw the key away after he turned the lock.

He did too many weird drugs in the 70s.
Both wings are flapping, but the bird is flying in circles.
In that brain of a wallet, there's nothing but pennies.

Her filament burnt out, oh dear.
She's not the swiftest deer in the forest.
If you look carefully, you can see between his ears.

The mall is open, but no one is shopping.
The lights are on, but nobody is home.
The only thing happening in that brain is popcorn popping.

# POST-STEM CELL TRANSPLANT: MEDICAL PERSPECTIVE

Getting through the first one hundred days after undergoing an autologous stem cell transplant is a tremendous benchmark. Olivia was exposed to a whopping dose of chemotherapy, designed to eliminate the bone marrow tissue where the myeloma cells live. New bone marrow stem cells were infused the day after the chemotherapy was finished to hasten the bone marrow function to recover and thereby reduce the risks of infection, low blood counts, and low platelet counts.

Most people feel nearly back to their usual selves by the time the one-hundred-day benchmark has passed, but there are a few lingering issues that may remain. Energy levels and prior exercise capacity may still not quite be back to pre-transplant levels for up to a few more months. Immunity is still suppressed for up to six months after transplant, and for this reason, prophylactic antiviral medications are continued. Cosmetic changes happen as well. When hair grows back on the head, it often comes back a different color (often darker or grayer) and with a different texture or shape (sometimes softer, sometimes curlier, or thicker). Nail beds are sensitive to chemotherapy and what patients will sometimes see are dark streaks in the nails that work themselves out over a long period of time. Skin changes are also apparent. The skin color may change to a darker tone (especially in people of color), and when the hair grows back on the face and chest, little pustules sometimes pop out as well, akin to teenage acne. Intellectual capacity and function can also take a brief hit after transplant. Work duties may seem especially burdensome, since thinking can seem to take some effort. ("Chemo-brain" is a very real phenomenon.)

I often tell my patients to expect 90 percent of pre-transplant global performance to be back and ready by one hundred days post-transplant. The remaining 10 percent takes the full six months to return. Usually by that time, the hair growth has come back with a vengeance, the lost weight has been regained, and people are back to playing tennis, jogging, or other exercise that they had enjoyed before.

At six months, some immune system function has returned, and we begin a series of vaccinations to replace the antibodies that were lost during the transplant process.

Below is the list and schedule of immunizations that are usually given post-stem cell transplant, bearing in mind that the list may be tailored to the particular situation that a patient may be in:

Post-Transplant Titer check and Immunization Schedule:

SIX MONTHS POST-TRANSPLANT:
1) Influenza vaccine (yearly)

2) Pneumococcal vaccine (every two months x four doses)

TWELVE MONTHS POST-TRANSPLANT:
1) Tetanus/Diptheria/Pertussis (every two months x three doses)

2) Hemophilus Influenza (every two months x three doses)

3) Inactivated Polio (every two months x three doses)

4) MMR (check titers first, and if negative, one dose only)

5) Hepatitis B (only if in selected population—usually health care workers)

6) Meningococcus Vaccine (once, only if in college or attending summer camp)

There are some long-term consequences and risks to stem cell transplant that should be noted. First of all, the exposure to the high-dose chemotherapy itself carries a long-term risk of secondary malignancies. The chemotherapy works by creating breaks in the DNA inside dividing cancer cells, leading to their early death. The chemotherapy can also create breaks in normally dividing cells in the body; these breaks can cause mutations in the genetic code that can lead to cancer later on in life. Although the risk is low, often quoted at 10 percent, people who undergo stem cell transplant are at higher risk for developing myelodysplastic syndrome (a disorganized and inefficient bone marrow space) or acute leukemia. These secondary malignancies show up years after the transplant and should be looked out for by the physician.

The second risk of transplant is that while most patients get their blood counts back (red and white blood cells, along with the platelets), a few do not have recovery within the first few weeks after the procedure. There are a subset of patients that will require transfusion for support for prolonged periods of time. Failure to fully recover blood counts tends to happen in patients who have been exposed to large amounts of chemotherapy or have undergone more than one transplant.

For the most part, however, the vast majority of patients do bounce back after transplant, with their disease in check. It takes time. When I talk about the transplant process with a patient, I often say to them, "You may like me now, but I know that there will come a time after transplant that you will hate me for taking away your energy and appetite. I know that there will come a time, however, that you will like me again and look back on the whole thing as something worth doing."

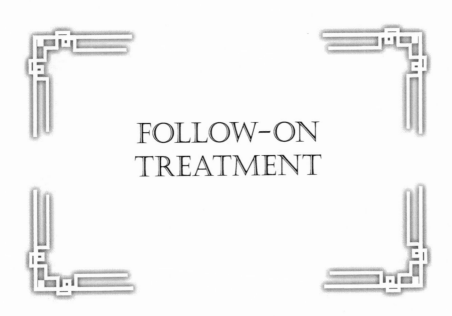

# FOLLOW-ON
# TREATMENT

From: Olivia Chin (oliviac@yahoo.com)    Sent: 08/28/09 2:01 PM
To: Friendlist
Cc:
Subject: A Village called Hope

Dear Friends,

I am packing up and getting ready to head home this Sunday. What a huge sense of relief. Going home! My family! My own bed! My kitchen! My space! Going from over 6,500 square feet to five hundred was an adjustment. Perhaps even more significant is that this studio, which I adore, was always considered a temporary dig.

*There's no place like home . . .*

Going home is a relief; however, there is a growing sense of anxiety of coping with everything and everybody. I haven't driven in over four months! I haven't really cooked anything in the same period of time. The stove in this studio has been turned on less than a half a dozen times in that period! Is my family going to expect too much? Will I repeat history and constantly overdo it? When Wai, Katie, and Elizabeth came last weekend, we didn't do much, but after they left I was exhausted for two days and napped. Rey and Lisette dropped by. Then Louise and Sal dropped by, and I expected to go to Soho afterward. Those plans were scrapped after their short visit even though the day was beautiful, warm, and dry. After seeing Dr. Mark on Thursday, I napped some more. Company is much loved but exhausting. I guess I need to practice moaning. When Wai and the kids are too much, I'll lay on the couch with the back of my hand on my forehead muttering, "uuooh" or "ooye" or even better yet, "je suis malade." With my luck, I'll fall asleep and mutter, "Hot pastrami on rye, not too fatty" or "The yellowtail sashimi, please."

*I'll get you, my pretty . . .*

It has taken me four months to come to terms mentally with the cancer diagnosis. I went from feeling as if I had been hit by a truck to now having an inner sense of calm. I will accept whatever life will hand me. As I've recently stated, I am living with myeloma. I am not dying of it.

I will beat the odds. With a large margin. There is no alternative, and I will not look back or to the side. That said, this was a rough week. I made three trips to Cornell Medical this week. I wish I could just have a year or even six months when I do not have to deal with any of this any more. It takes an enormous amount of mental discipline to keep away from the dark side.

*I'm melting . . .*

Physically, I still limp a bit, but I can walk. My hair is coming in—I graduated from baby cactus to Velveteen Rabbit. I have sharp pains between the shoulders. My eyes are still funky, as is my skin. I get tired easily, and there is no second wind. But I feel so much better than before the stem cell transplant. In comparison, I feel fantastic! Fabulous! The next step for me is chemo. There appear to be two camps in the medical field. There are doctors who feel if you are doing well, to leave well enough alone. There are doctors who feel the data they have indicates one does better on some regimen. In my case, we're not taking any chances due to the extra twist of amyloidosis. Next week, I start a new regimen of oral chemo, Revlimid. With luck, it will prolong the good times ahead, which will be put to full use enjoying my family and friends. (Did I neglect to mention food?)

*Scarecrows don't talk, do they???*

Spiritually, I am soaring in the sky. My faith has grown, and I have learned to accept that which cannot be rationalized and that which cannot be explained. I have learned to accept what once was unacceptable with grace. When one considers all that has happened . . . you could focus on the negative. We spent gobs of money on medical expenses this year. We are still in jeopardy of losing our source of income. Our savings has declined. The massive layoffs in our area means our community will be hard hit and homes will not sell well for years to come. Friends and colleagues have been impacted. My mother hurt herself twice badly in the last year. A very close friend of ours was also diagnosed with myeloma, and she is recovering from her transplant too. And the list goes on. Just looking at this city and all the empty storefronts and offices can be depressing.

*I am the great and powerful . . .*

But, we were able to switch insurance companies just when we needed. We happened unknowingly upon a world-class myeloma clinic for a second opinion. We got a corrected and amended diagnosis in a short period of time. Had the medical team upstate diagnosed multiple myeloma, it is unlikely that they would found amyloidosis. The stem cell treatment was fine, all things considered. The night in the hospital when I thought I was going to give up, a night nurse came in to check; he was one beautiful male specimen. I laughed, thinking that they scheduled him in when needed. Hope Lodge was amazing. Then the studio opened up just as we needed it. Wai managed to hold everybody together, and he even brought me bedside *NY Times* and café lattes. We met wonderful people along the way. We made new friends. We renewed ties with old friends. Our friends, family, and a support system we did not know we had were there for us, waiting in the wings. Our children visited several friends' homes in our area, the Thousand Islands, the Chesapeake Bay, the Poconos, Queens, Long Island, Skaneateles, and they are at a private lake in PA right now with my friend Judith. Our children grew along the way and got to really know many of our friends and my brother. Our dog was cared for and loved by another family for much of the year. I am going home to be with loved ones. I missed them so.

*These slippers will take you home . . .*

Dr. Tomer Mark is collaborating with me on a book. He is providing the medical perspective, the straight man in this comedy team. (Did you know he challenged me to figure out his e-mail? He actually tossed the gauntlet! So I figured out the e-mail userid codes at Cornell Medical and started bombarding his inbox.) He can be very funny, but for the most part, maintains a very professional decorum. He is an extremely capable and intelligent doctor, but even more important, as I get to know him better, he is a really good man. He has earned my respect. And he eats sushi!

*I hereby confer upon you the honorary degree of ThD . . .*

It takes a village. My village is called Hope.

*Hold onto your hope.*

*Love,*
*Olivia*

PS: Scientists report that fish and other ocean wildlife are starting to mysteriously disappear from the Pacific too. Here fishy, fishy, fishy! Here fishy, fishy!

From: Olivia Chin (oliviac@yahoo.com)     Sent: 09/18/09 10:12 AM
To: Friendlist
Cc:
Subject: Pain and Fear

Dear Friends,

First of all, it took a week to get my e-mail back up, and a few more days before I was able to clean up the e-mails from the transition from laptop to desktop. It goes without saying that the first order of business was checking out the jokes!

Michael said it sucked that he lost his playmate in New York City. Well, it sucks even more to lose a playmate and the whole playground! I have been at home for two weeks now. The return home was rather disappointing—I came home with excruciating pain in the shoulder. About twenty minutes into the four-hour car ride home, I knew I was in trouble. So I have been sleeping. I am not sure if the pain is due to the packing and moving or if it is the amyloidosis rearing its ugly head or if it is the neuropathy getting the best of me while the nerves are jangling around. The pain was pretty intense. It's getting a little better. The return from solitude to a full week with kids at home was tough. If I had to do it over again, I would either have come home after the kids started school, or I would have come home while having the kids hang out elsewhere for the week. Although I love being with the girls, it was a bit much to come home to . . . I just wish I were in better shape. Pain and fear sure put a damper on everything.

I started taking the chemo that hopefully will prolong remission or partial remission. It makes me tired. It is supposed to cause gastric distress—none in my case, of course! It comes with a number of side effects, but the main ones for me are fatigue, swelling of feet, and loud heart beats. It also can cause low blood counts, possibly a lower immune system. I have been thinking about the 550-plus cases of swine flu at Cornell University. My heart goes out to the parents of the one twenty-year-old who died.

Last Wednesday, school started for Katie and Elizabeth. My kids went squealing into the building once they realized that the annual Happy

Feet dance was taking place right outside the school by the bus drop off! Every year, I do the Happy Feet dance on the first day of school—much to their merriment and embarrassment. A couple of years ago, a departing principal did the reciprocating Happy Feet dance on the last day of school! They are both busy already with homework. Elizabeth started middle school this year. It starts a year earlier in their school. It is a good thing, though—they are exposed to middle school teachers who have specialized training in their field. The teachers are all passionate about the subject matter they teach. The girls have grown up this summer. The other morning while getting ready for school, Elizabeth accidentally dropped a heavy can on her foot. She was in a lot of pain, but she did not make a peep. Katie came by to comfort her, neither one of them making a sound to alert me that there was anything amiss. When I saw the two of them together, I realized that not only were they trying hard to hide the pain, but that Katie had taken on a mothering role. I felt really bad at first—only to realize that they are supporting each other rather than vying for attention. What an incredible journey!

Wai has been busy getting everything done that usually takes both of us to do. When I first got home, Wai said to me that if cooking was too much, that we could eat out or—GASP—he could cook. I responded with, "Who is she?!" One has to understand that in twenty-seven years of marriage, he has expected a hot meal, every night. Then one evening, when I was worn out, he volunteered to finish cooking dinner. I responded with "What is her name?!!" The funniest event however was on Labor Day. Elizabeth decided to make me French toast as a surprise for breakfast, so she woke Wai up at 5:30 a.m. to get breakfast going!

As the day wears on, I wear out, so I have been marinating meats and veggies, and Wai grills. Gervlyne dropped off this wicked Haitian dish called legume, and Ann Marie came by with pizza and wings. I can't thank you all enough—all of you who are either cooking or planning on having food delivered. Okay, I got the message—my village wants to help! On Tuesdays, Wednesdays, and Thursdays, Wai or I pick up the kids from school and take them to dance class. By the time we get home, it's hard to whip something together. If you want to drop something off at school at three p.m., it would be lovely. (Choke!) It is really hard to accept help. Nicole finally convinced me that she would ask me for help if she needed it and to get off my duff, swallow my pride, and ask for help. Since Katie cannot have wheat, dairy, or eggs, which makes it that much harder to ask for help, all I can suggest is spiedies (a local specialty), pizza, and wings (she eats the wings), chili, and anything with meat, potatoes, corn, quinoa, barley, and rice. Help is nice—on the other hand, just your company would be wonderful.

*Love,*
*Olivia*

From: Olivia Chin (oliviac@yahoo.com)    Sent: 09/18/09 11:49 AM
To: "Nick You"
Cc:
Subject: Pain

Dear Nicky,

I am sick and tired of being sick and tired.

It would be so nice to just have a few days completely free of all these trappings. I went to see my family physician; I went to get a CT scan; I went to see the local hematologist. I go back again this afternoon for another blood test.

This is my new life. I hate my new life.

Perhaps the chemo is what is dragging me down. I am so tired. I take naps. The shoulder pain is getting to me. At the best of times, it feels like incredibly bad sunburn. At the worst of times, it feels as if I have razor blades in my shoulder. Pain does not help my disposition. For a week, I was able to keep the nasty side of me away. Now the sharks are back!

My friends are cooking. We have had legume, rice and beans, pizza and wings, macaroni and cheese, salad, and a rice pasta dish. I cannot believe how much people want to help. Food is the easiest way for people to show us how much they care. I accept it because I don't know what else to do. Come plant my fall mums for me? Come weed the yard that got overgrown this summer? Clean out my donation pile of stuff and bring it to the mission? That's the help I really need. Maybe I will ask.

Love,
Olivia

From: nicole                                    Sent: 09/19/09 11:49 AM
To: "olivia chin"
Cc:
Subject: You're all mine, O! Well, at least today, that is!

O,

I'm bringing food to school at three p.m. today. Keep your fingers crossed.
Why, you ask? Because the other day when I was cooking, the boys called
out, "What's that horrible smell?!" To which I replied simply, "Dinner."

Don't worry, though. I'll bring a bar of Swiss chocolate. Just in case . . .

Nicole

From: Olivia Chin (oliviac@yahoo.com) Sent: 09/21/09 3:11 PM
To: "Nick You"
Cc:
Subject: Thinking

Dear Nicky,

I just heard from a fellow myeloma patient—it is really sad. She has had two stem cell transplants, her myeloma is back, and her doctor in Syracuse has just told her there is nothing else she can do.

There has to be another way. I recommended she go to Dr. Niesvizky as well as Dr. Lionel, another doctor who does extensive clinical trials. There has to be something—any type of treatment. She has had a broken hip as well as a broken rib recently. And yet they tell her she has no bone lesions. Why can't there be any treatment left for her? Or is it that there is no treatment left from her doctor in Syracuse?

When I first received the diagnosis and my treatment was going to be the autologous stem cell transplant, I was concerned. Everyone else seemed to be going under some form of chemotherapy prior to the stem cell transplant. Due to the amyloidosis, it was understood that my treatment was going to be aggressive. So we did a stem cell rather quickly. When you stop to think about it, a stem cell transplant is really rather amazing. It is sort of like rebooting a PC. You reboot yourself and hope for the best. Some people have a long time before needing another reboot, some people don't respond at all. I hope I have a long time, but even if I don't, I was lucky to be in good enough shape to be able to have a transplant. Many people are not well enough to have a transplant. In the case of this patient, she is no longer well enough for a third transplant. Why did they wait so long?

Since the stem cell, I am taking Revlimid. There are two major choices in today's world of myeloma post-transplant: those who feel that they should leave well enough alone and those who feel some maintenance treatment is needed. This other lady was on nothing. Who knows if she would have been better off on Revlimid or Thalidomide? Now she feels as if her back is against the wall, looking for anything that will prolong her life. Her stem cell options have run out. As scared as I get sometimes, there must be nothing as frightening as hearing from your doctor that there is no more treatment. Should she have been on something? Would it have not made any difference?

How terrifying is it to realize that there are no remaining options? How frightening is it to be without any choices? I hope I will have the courage to face the inevitable when the time comes. I hope I will be able to keep my faith. I hope I will be strong enough to deal with the pain. Perhaps I will allow myself to cry a little bit from time to time—but only a tiny little bit. This much I know—life will continue even after it seems too hard. And it will be alright.

There are people who live an easy life, with few problems, much happiness, and a painless end. There are people who live an existence that is unbelievably difficult, with much harshness and suffering. Sometimes I wonder what twists our lives take, what choices make our lives so very different? What if, based on certain factors, we end up with different endings to our lives? As much as I would have preferred to not have multiple myeloma and amyloidosis, I am a product of these diseases now. Life is not going to be a straight line anymore. And it will be alright.

Perhaps my future will be like this patient, with myeloma rearing it's head shortly. Or perhaps my future will have myeloma in the far distance. Or perhaps by the time it comes around, there will be a cure. Either way, life goes on. And it will be alright.

Love,
Olivia

# FOLLOW-ON TREATMENT: MEDICAL PERSPECTIVE

There are still lingering questions and issues that remain after recovery from stem cell transplant occurs, such as:

- I know that stem cell transplant is not a cure for myeloma; when can I expect it to come back?
- Is it necessary to go through a second transplant (tandem)—will it make me live longer?
- Do I need any further chemotherapy after a transplant, or do we watch-and-wait?
- How long are my cryopreserved stem cells good for?

All of the above questions are valid. Traditionally, no chemotherapy is given after autologous stem cell transplant for myeloma. The average time until progression of disease (meaning, time needed until a new treatment for myeloma relapse after transplant) ranged anywhere from between twenty-four to thirty-six months. Many factors play into the time until relapse, but perhaps the most important is the quality of the disease response prior to and following the transplant; simply put, the more disease that is eradicated prior to and by the transplant, the longer the post-transplant remission lasts. Persons who achieve a complete remission prior to transplant, or achieve one with the help of transplant, do the best overall, in terms of length of time needed until the next treatment is necessary.

There have been several clinical trials that have looked at extending the duration of remission after autologous stem cell transplant in myeloma using a variety of strategies. One technique is to perform two transplants back to back, in a method called a tandem transplant. In this case, a standard stem cell transplant is performed and when recovery from the first occurs, usually at around one hundred days, another stem cell transplant, the second, is done. Very high rates of complete remission are achieved using this technique, and it has been shown in a trial where patients are randomized to either one or two transplants that statistically the patients in the two-transplant arm live longer. As one could imagine, there was greater overall toxicity from two transplants; overall time to recovery was twice as long, and there were twice as many opportunities for infections and other complications. A critical look at the results, however, revealed an interesting finding: only those patients who had achieved less than a 90 percent reduction in myeloma burden with the first transplant actually derived any benefit from undergoing the second one! One way to look at this is that the second transplant "rescued" incomplete responders to the first; another view is that people who achieved a good response to the transplant do not necessarily need to be exposed to the potential toxicities of another one. For this reason, in most medical centers, tandem transplants are not planned *a priori* (although there are notable exceptions to this treatment philosophy); but rather, a second transplant is usually offered when the response is assessed after the first transplant is complete. If the stem cells were collected and cryopreserved properly, they will remain functional for many years; I myself have used cells collected fifteen years ago for a first transplant to do a second transplant at relapse. There is no clock running out on the cells per se, therefore, the stem cell viability should not be a major issue when deciding when/whether to undergo a second transplant.

When the transplant is complete and recovery has occurred, most people can go back to work and living their lives as before, but there are lingering thoughts of when the myeloma will return. Traditionally, most oncologists and patients took a watch-and-wait approach for after-transplant care, believing that the myeloma could be treated effectively when it returned and that early intervention would not lead to a longer lifespan but rather would only prolong the time that the patient needed to be on chemotherapy in a sort of lead-time bias. Recently reported trials of patients with myeloma randomized post-transplant to either a placebo or thalidomide show a distinct overall survival benefit for the thalidomide arm. Newer studies are being conducted and early reports show similar benefits for dosing either bortezomib or lenalidomide post-transplant as well. While maintenance therapy post-transplant is gaining in popularity, there are still some caveats. Do the long-term use of these treatments have any side effects, like secondary malignancies? We already know that prolonged use of some older chemotherapeutics, like melphalan, can damage the bone marrow and lead to myelodysplastic syndrome and leukemia. Thalidomide, bortezomib, and lenalidomide have not been in clinical use for myeloma for a long period of time and this question remains to be answered. Another question to be asked is whether the known side effects of these drugs, such as peripheral neuropathy or somnolence, can be tolerated for the long periods of time needed (on the scale of years) to show the survival benefit. In the end, the choice of maintenance therapy post-transplant should be discussed with all of the pros and cons presented objectively.

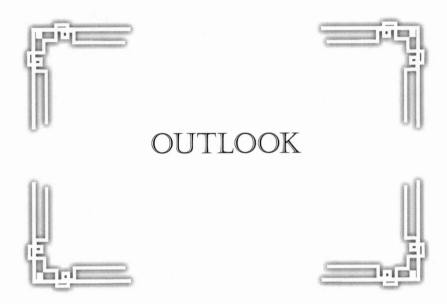

OUTLOOK

From: Olivia Chin (oliviac@yahoo.com)    Sent: 10/13/09 11:17 AM
To: Friendlist
Cc:
Subject: Funky Fingernails

Dear Friends,

Hi everyone!

The end of my fingernails are discoloured due to the major chemotherapy
way back at the beginning of the stem cell transplant. The colour
has moved to the tips of my nails now. In another month or so, the
discoloration will be gone. It feels as if my nails symbolize everything
that has happened! Slowly but surely, the poison that was in me is now
leaving. I can do much more now with only a few restrictions. There is
nothing I cannot eat. I have recently started another chemo that should
keep me healthier for a longer time. That is a careful way of saying that
we would really like this chemo to keep the big stuff at bay! It has some
strange side effects. Fatigue is the first one. I sleep and sleep and sleep.
The second one is the sound of my own heart beating. The third one is
odd—I cannot seem to talk sometimes. A friend of mine said at lunch
the other day that she likes me this way. She says I seem more thoughtful
about what I want to say.

*Ya think?*

Well, I am happy to say that the pain in the shoulders has lessened
significantly! It took about two months for the pain to lessen. When the
pain started to stop, I finally looked around myself and freaked. This place
has not been cleaned for over three years! There is stuff everywhere! So I
started cleaning up—sometimes a few minutes a day, sometimes an hour a
day. I have been taking stuff to the Salvation Army. It will take me months
to sort through everything. I am happy to say I can see the floor again in
the living room and dining room. And then I realized that, just like this
house, my life got to be a real mess too. So now I try to spend time with
the girls, baking or scrapbooking or whatever it is they want to do for
fun. If they want a sleepover or go to a Fall Festival, they can.

*How did it get so bad?*

I just got back from seeing Dr. Mark. My last set of lab tests was rather significant because they were the first ones after the new chemo. They were good! Until now, the lab results were alright, but they were creeping up. This new set of results shows some significant reductions where we want reductions. I am very happy. (Who cares if I can't talk? I'll just e-mail instead!) Michael and I met in NYC for a great time. (Hm? Oh, we ate mussels and a fondue at Artisanal). Then Wai and the kids came down to bring me back up. The kids got to try the 2nd Ave Deli, where they enjoyed their meal—but relished the four chocolate soda chasers at the end! (Normally, you get one). The waiter and waitress kept them coming at the end of the meal! We rushed back from NYC because Elizabeth was a flower girl at a very special wedding. The wedding was wonderful! It was the best ever! It was touching. It was fun. The food was fabulous. I did the centerpieces, which turned out rather nice. Elizabeth did what she was supposed to do, which was to look really cute. What was really special was that we have watched the bride grow up from infancy into a beautiful young woman, both inside and outside. Also touching is that the bride's mother, Sally, went through a stem cell transplant about twenty days before me. We have supported each other. At one point, she and I danced to a special song, the significance of which was only for her and me: "I will survive."

*Disco duck!*

What comes next is chemo until the end of the good times. I am to take this chemo called Revlimid or lenalidomide until the myeloma and amyloidosis come back aggressively. I always said there was no cure, just treatment for now. That means the myeloma will grow at some point. It doesn't matter to me at this point when it grows; all I know is, I am enjoying life for now. I am enjoying my girls for now. I am hounding Wai for now.

*Life is good.*

So my outlook is positive. I would like to thank all of you who came through with gifts of food. There was a period when I was in terrible pain, and it really helped. This is the first year my Halloween decorations are up before Halloween. I hope to take them down within a few days afterward too! I plan to enjoy my Christmas this year as well. You know you are getting older when you think about the tree and all the trimmings and the four-letter words that go with it make "Bah humbug" seem merry. Well this year, it's going to be a good one!

*Love,*
*Olivia*

From: Olivia Chin (oliviac@yahoo.com)     Sent: 10/31/09 11:29 AM
To: Friendlist
Cc:
Subject: Shark Costume and Blueberry Pie

Hi everyone!

It has been an incredible sequence of events since I last wrote. First of all,
on Monday two weeks ago, I started cutting out and pinning Elizabeth's
Halloween costume. She wanted to be a shark. Last year, had she asked,
I would have howled at her along the lines of "I'm in too much pain to
sew you a &*#@$%!! shark costume!" Two years ago, I would have yelled,
"Are you nuts? Can you not just buy a witch or alien costume? I'm too
busy teaching technology and running around on various committees!"
This year, I smiled benignly at her and said, "Sure, darling! We'll make
you a shark costume!" So off to the fabric store we go. No shark pattern.
So off I go to the Open Door Mission and the Salvation Army. I find
a pattern! It only goes up to size six. I figure I can make it larger for
her—she's a very small ten anyway.

*Cut. Cut. Pin. Pin. Baste.*

The last week I was back down to NYC, I was there to see a retinologist,
to get a regular flu shot, and to get a MRI of the head. I went to see the
retinologist, who has Nurse Bumble Fingers on his staff. She tried to get
the dye into me and failed after five times. So I have to go back next week
for them to try again! Then I got my shot from Dr. Mark in a retrofitted
bathroom made to look like a throne room set up just for flu shots. Very
weird. I finally went for my MRI, and they were delayed. But I stayed; by
that time, my eyes were dilated and I had holes all over from the attempts
at the dye insertion. They get an IV in on the first try. Then I went to eat
with friends. The restaurant was so noisy, I never heard my cell phone
ring, so I didn't get the message from Dr. Mark until later. It essentially
said to please stay in NY because the MRI was bad. It showed a mostly
blocked left carotid in the head. I call and leave messages for friends who
were coming to our house on Friday to say it isn't a good time.

*So, Priceline it was.*

The next morning, I call Dr. Mark, and he said he would try to get me an appointment with a neurosurgeon. He called back less than two hours later with an appointment at three p.m. with Dr. Athos Patsalides. I had most of the day to fool around in NYC. Sweet! Well, I had some banking issues to do, and then, it was lunchtime. I decided to go to an upscale restaurant and order the most decadent food I could, since going to see a neurosurgeon after an MRI of the brain could hardly forebode good news. Off to the Morgan Museum I went, where they have a delightful restaurant, the type where the waiter comes with the bread tray and asks you if you would like the multi-grain roll, the French sourdough boule, or the olive-and-salt twist. All three please. (I left the multi-grain—too healthy). I had an absolutely fabulous lobster salad with watercress, followed by a crème leche cake, not too sweet. Lunch having taken over one and a half hours, I sadly realize there is no time left to see anything at the museum. So off I go to see this Dr. Patsalides. I get there. He sends notice and apologizes, he is late. I wait. He comes. He explains, showing me on the MRI, that there are five to seven strokes, two larger ones, the rest smaller, possibly TIAs. He explains that the carotid is over 95 percent blocked and asks me if I have had any other symptoms besides not being able to talk. Any weakness in the right hand? No. Any weakness in the right foot or leg? No. Any dizziness? No. Any balance issues? No. And I am thinking: *I DON'T TALK ALL THE TIME! HOW OFTEN ARE THESE DAMN THINGS HAPPENING?* It is now nearly five p.m. He looks at his calendar, thinks a bit, and then asks me if I can stay in NY for the night. He could do an angiogram the next day.

*Out of my way, doc. I need access to your PC to get my hotel!*

So the next day, he does the angiogram. They go in through your groin and into an artery and snake up to your head. Then they inject dye at various times and sync it to an MRI machine that takes pictures at all angles. The doctor tells me it is not a clot and that he will call me Monday afternoon after he has a conference with other doctors to figure out what to do. It might be aggressive medical therapy and/or a stent. (I am glad I had the lobster salad). Wai comes down to get me out of there and take me home. We get home very late; it is raining. I get into the house. I take off my coat. Then the pain hits. The pain is so intense I cannot speak for an entirely different reason. Wai is trying to go to bed, and I manage to tell him to stick around in case I have to go to the ER. When I can finally talk, I realize my entire right leg is now swollen and as hard as a rock. I try to reach the doctor, but his messaging system is not working. I try to reach his nurse, same number. I finally call another doctor in the same office (the guy who did the biopsy on the ankle six months ago). The messaging service picks up, the doctor on call will call back. I wait, in incredible pain. The friends who were called two nights before are banging on the door. I hobble over, and in thirty seconds, they realize there has been a mistake and that there is possibly a medical emergency happening. They leave for a hotel. Suddenly, the pain stops. The hardness is subsiding. The phone rings. The doctor on call says not to worry, as long as the site is not bleeding profusely, I should be fine. Call back if it happens again and go to an ER.

*No—methinks go to an ER and then possibly call.*

The next morning, Saturday morning, I wake up feeling sore, but fine. I suddenly realize that the Halloween party is tonight! The sewing machine and all the bits come downstairs. At 8:30 a.m., I am sitting with my right leg extended on the pedal, sewing like mad. Katie is coughing. Wai and the kids leave for shopping. I am sitting in the weirdest position, with the machine going strong. Midmorning, I am sewing and stuffing the large tail and fin. Late morning, Sally pops by to return some hats she had borrowed. (I collect hats from the forties.) She starts hand sewing. The family comes back. We eat lunch. Sally and I are still sewing. Early afternoon, the costume is done! It is glorious! The jumpsuit has an attached tail and fin! The headpiece has great white, sparkling teeth! Sally leaves. The kids get ready for the school party. Wai and I enjoy some Mexican food. By the time the meal is over, I am so tired, but happy. We go to pick up the kids. They are tired. They sleep with me. Katie coughs.

*Life is good, right?*

Sunday morning, Katie wakes up burning hot. 103.6° F. Wai is gone to the Ithaca book sale. I am giving her Tylenol when Judith calls to tell me about her week. Her two grandsons had H1N1. She watched them so their newborn sister would be safe. I hang up. I am thinking. It doesn't take long. Face mask on, I drag Katie to the walk-in clinic. Most likely H1N1, they give both of us Tamiflu. The walk-in doctor is freaking out because of my suppressed immunity. The pharmacies in Owego say they do not have Tamiflu in the dosage prescribed for Katie. Back to the walk-in, can she take mine? No. Back to the pharmacy, I tell them to make the damn dosage using adult capsules in a suspension for her. We get home; we segregate to different parts of the house. She has a child face mask from the walk-in. I have mine on. Wai comes home. What's for dinner?

*Oh, Lord.*

Monday night, Dr. Mark is in town to give a talk about Revlimid to Broome Oncology, something I initiated months ago. Rather than stay at home, I leave for the restaurant so Katie can have the run of the house without her face mask. I had dinner by myself in the restaurant, waiting for Dr. Mark. He shows up after his discussion. I inform him about the swine flu on top of the angiogram. I tell him the book has more chapters to come . . . possibly a sequel. He says he is glad the book was not immediately over.

*Ha!*

So now, finally, at the end of the week, I sit back to relax. Friends dropped off an incredible blueberry pie, which I am finishing with my coffee. It is the weekend, and Wai has taken the kids out again. Katie returned to school earlier this week. She is over her fever and her medications. I am still on Tamiflu. In ten days, I am going to have a stent put in my brain. And I realize that this is the first time this year that I have not even thought about myeloma or amyloidosis.

*Life goes on.*

No matter what happens, no matter how serious or tragic the event, life goes on. There is always tomorrow, there is always another day. There is always another blueberry pie.

*Love,*
*Olivia*

# HOLIDAY NEWSLETTER 2009

What a year it has been! After a year of trying to get a correct medical diagnosis locally for pain in my leg and foot, I went to Weill-Cornell in NYC. Early spring, I was diagnosed with amyloidosis, followed quickly with an additional diagnosis of multiple myeloma. Given the rampant nature of amyloidosis and its fairly fast decimation rate, I was admitted almost immediately for a stem cell transplant. By early May, I was in Cornell/New York Presbyterian Hospital. The hospital was amazing, with a staff that never quit. By early June, I was out, bald as a cucumber, weak as a caterpillar. I stayed at the American Cancer Society Hope Lodge NYC for two weeks, and then moved into a studio in NYC that friends had available. I stayed in NYC for four months to be in a very clean environment and to be able to see my doctors on a regular basis. I owe it all to my doctors, Dr. Niesvizky and Dr. Mark. Dr. Mark will always have a special place in my heart—he lent me his Nintendo DS (which he plays during his commute to work) through the entire stem cell transplant! Although most of the time I was too tired to play, his supreme sacrifice was well noted.

In the meantime, Katie and Elizabeth got fantastic report cards. They also danced in competitions, where they did very well. Summer vacation began, with the kids going to friends all over the East coast. They stayed with friends from the Chesapeake Bay to Skaneateles, from Long Island to a lake in Pennsylvania. For ten weeks, Katie and Elizabeth went from home to home, cottage to cottage, except for two weeks, which they spent with their uncle in Owego. It was a growing experience for them, dealing with excitement and fun, homesickness and fear. In the meantime, Wai was running back and forth from Owego to NYC. Wai was a pillar of strength through it all.

Our family regrouped in the beginning of September. The girls and I came home. Elizabeth started middle school in fifth grade, Katie started seventh grade. They returned to school several years more mature than when school let out for the summer. One morning, Elizabeth hurt herself, but she kept her tears silent so as not to bother me. Katie came around and started comforting her quietly. It wasn't until I found them huddled together that I realized the bond they had formed while I was away, taking care of each other, depending on each other. I was moved to tears. And so we are together. Healing. Repairing. Hoping. A stem cell transplant doesn't cure what I have, but it buys time. After I came home, friends dropped off gifts of food. Between the care the girls received over the summer, the sharing, the praying, and the gifts of food, all I can say is that a stem cell transplant takes a village. And what a fabulous village I have! *My village rocks!*

The kids are still dancing. They danced the *Russian Nutcracker* with the Moscow Ballet, and they just finished the *Russian Nutcracker* with Rafael Grigorian. Elizabeth got the coveted role of the Nutcracker this year! Katie is starting Science Olympiad. Wai is working still. I am mostly at home—no more volunteer work for me! I take the kids where they need to go, and I cook—and that's about it. In addition, Katie came down with H1N1, and I caught strep throat! With my weakened immune system, Katie and I spent a week in this house mostly segregated, wearing face masks! I still go to NYC regularly for follow-up appointments with Dr. Mark, but the trips accelerated when an MRI of the head came back positive for a carotid obstruction. The level of care I've received at Cornell is amazing. Two days after the MRI, I had an angiogram. Since then, I've been down for an intercranial stent and laser retinal surgery. Sigh. So many rich, smart, handsome men! Sigh. Too bad they're all doctors . . .

Apart from this all-consuming string of medical events, there is more . . . I've decided to slowly clean out the house. Those of you who have seen this place realize that it is a project that will take years! So I can't figure out if I am mildly depressed because of the medical stuff that won't quit, or whether it is a good thing to divert me from the endless task of cleaning. I did just decide however to quit rushing during the trips downstate and to spend some time enjoying myself, either visiting friends or gong to museums—or stopping by La Maison du Chocolat. Now *that* is a place that will lift my spirits! Speaking of the spirit, my faith continues to grow, in spite of the illness, and not because of it. I've been touched deeply in many ways this last year. There is more to faith than I could ever want to believe!

Here's hoping that your holiday season brings you good spirits and health!

Love,
Olivia

Hi, Helene!

We got back from China last week, and all four of us were sick. We walked into the plane for the trip home with colds, and we walked out of that same plane really sick. We hit the walk-in clinic before even going home. We all had pneumonia! Otherwise, all is fine. The kids started school on Wednesday. Elizabeth transitioned from Catholic to public school this year. She started at the Owego Middle School in sixth grade. She loves her new school! Katie started eighth grade, still at the private school. Then I was down in NYC last Wednesday and Thursday with my mom (aargh!) for business, and I also did my medical appointments.

*She drives me nuts.*

The steroids are working! Steroids enhance the effectiveness of the chemotherapy. Even though it makes me feel like I am in a 24/7 hot flash (along with one day a week when I feel like the baby in *The Incredibles* who flames up), after six weeks of steroids, my numbers are down. This is a good thing, considering they had been climbing for four to five months, and my doctor was getting concerned. The steroids are supposed to make me gain weight, but so far I've lost five pounds and that's with eating everything in sight in China. Oh the food! We had dumplings, noodles, xiao long bao (mostly pork, but a few with hairy crab roe), hot pot, roast duck, stir-fries, Muslim food, Japanese udon, and I, of course, ate every street food I could find. Katie joined me. We had great street food, all of it very fresh. Wai and Elizabeth were too chicken to eat off the street vendors.

I am off to Boston to see Dr. Comenzo next week. He is a leading amyloidosis specialist. Mary is driving. Her goal is to eat well while there. Mine is to follow her lead. We're staying with an old friend from NYU. He was the assistant professor in the chemistry department. He was the older brother of a Chinese colleague of my father's, and his job was to be my chaperone. We hung out a lot during my freshman year, sightseeing, eating, and shopping. It was all very platonic. However, word got back to my parents that I was spending a lot of time with this somewhat older guy. Anyway, he lived in an upscale rooming house in Manhattan, with minimal cooking facilities. He was dying to cook, and he asked me if he could use my kitchen in my apartment in Queens. So he did his shopping and came over and cooked this incredible meal. As we finished eating, a pair of familiar shoes started coming down my stairs. It was my mother, unannounced from Switzerland, coming to check on me. You can imagine how it looked. I should have changed the locks.

*She drives me nuts.*

I'm going to be in NYC in October and would love to stay with you. Finally being on my own again. The last four trips involved my kids, and then Wai, and then the entire family, and then my mom. The one with the kids was interesting—we arrived in NY the day it hit 103°F in Central Park. I took them to a Belgium bistro for really good mussels. They said it was the best food they ever had. But did we sweat on the way there and back to the hospital! The next trip, I went down for eye surgery, and Wai and I stayed in Secaucus. (We didn't think you would have wanted us to bug you leaving for the hospital at five a.m.) That was interesting. The doctor, Dr. Chan, was initially convinced it was diabetic in nature. I disgreed with him, but since I couldn't see out of my left eye, I really had no choice. They went in and found out it was something totally different, related to blood clotting. At which point (I was semi-conscious by then), I blurted out, "I told you it wasn't diabetic retinopathy!" They were just a little surprised that I was listening and able to talk! They fixed what they could. During China, my sight came back—blurry and distorted, but back. Last week, they were amazed how much vision came back to my left eye. I think another month off somewhere would be good. No cooking. No cleaning. No anything but sightseeing, shopping, and eating. Then on the way to China, we all stayed at Secaucus, NJ (left from Newark), and I took the bus into Manhattan with Katie. And then, this last trip with my mom.

*She drives me nuts.*

I swear the stress of not taking good care of her is so much less stressful than being with her. I used to take her out about two to three times a week. Now I see her about once every one to two weeks, and I try to be with my family when possible. (She behaves differently with other people around). She can take a cab to the big grocery store (very cheap), and she walks to the small grocery, pharmacy, and shops in Owego. But the mind games that only mothers can play with daughters are now reduced to a minimum. It feels very selfish, but after all that's happened, I just can't take the stress anymore. On our last trip to NY together, she started picking as soon as she got into my car. It's funny how you can love someone so much, but then in the midst of trouble, the stress of being with that person can drive you over the edge. I always thought I would want to be with my mother a lot if anything crummy ever happened to me.

*She drives me nuts.*

We had a great trip in China. Beijing makes NYC look like a small dump. There are very few hutongs left. Everything is newly developed, everything is clean, everything is so modern. Xian used to be a sleepy town, but no more! Huge malls everywhere! Lots of restaurants, shops, and huge grocery stores! The terracotta soldier complex has been much developed since our last visit. Guilin was beautiful. The mountain and river scenes were spectacular. We also saw several other things there: an underground cave and a minority village, just to name a few. Guilin used to be a one-street village. Now it has grown, and they are building a whole new high-rise addition on the outskirts of the city. I'm not sure if it's due to city planning or due to foundations for taller buildings not being able to be built in the older section of town. Hangzhou was really nice. There are no high-rises right on the lake. The scale of the city was very livable, with some city planning that made it all work. And last, we were in Shanghai. We stayed in this apartment hotel right smack in the middle of restaurant row. By that time, we were done shopping, we were done sightseeing, and we were beginning to get sick. Toan met us there with Matthew! His wife had this trip planned to Shanghai about six months ago, a big international meeting for her work. So Toan came up and stayed for three days. We ate. We hung out. We had a good time.

Love,
Olivia

# OUTLOOK:
# MEDICAL PERSPECTIVE

Olivia has been through a whirlwind of life-changing events throughout the past year, starting with a diagnosis of cancer, through stem cell transplant, and now on maintenance chemotherapy. She knows that she still has myeloma, but her outlook has the grim determination of a survivor. She is justified in being optimistic about her long-term prospects given the advances in myeloma made over the last decade. When I went to medical school, I was taught that myeloma was a universally fatal malignancy, with an average survival of three years. Drugs such as melphalan and prednisone, when given in low doses, could produce favorable disease responses in about 50 percent of the patients, but did not lead to any increase in overall survival. The advent of high-dose chemotherapy with autologous stem cell support was the first therapy shown to improve survival in a randomized trial, and it became the new standard of care; however, the lifespan improvement averaged at slightly less than one year.

The introduction of the "novel agents" in myeloma produced a sea change that has provided hope for thousands of patients. Bortezomib, thalidomide, and lenalidomide have all been shown to improve overall survival for relapsed myeloma. All of these agents can be tolerated and used for long periods of time, leading to longer durations of remission during maintenance therapy. Although we are still working in the myeloma community to determine the optimal dosing strategy and combination of these drugs, the overall survival for the younger patient with myeloma has improved tremendously, from three years to eight years. Newly diagnosed patients with good-risk disease may now expect to live a decade, on average.

A new generation of drug therapy for myeloma is under development and currently in clinical trials. A novel proteasome inhibitor call Carfilzomib with a different target of action than bortezomib has shown some promise. The main advantage of carfilzomib is that it does not seem to carry the same risk of causing peripheral neuropathy that bortezomib does, although it remains to be seen if it is as effective an anti-myeloma therapy. The next immunomodulatory drug called Pomalidomide is also currently being tested. The side effect profile seems to be similar to lenalidomide, in that it may lead to low blood counts and increased risk of clotting. Excitingly, it appears that about 50 percent of people who do not respond favorable any longer to lenalidomide will get good results with pomalidomide.

Other targets of therapy are also under investigation, including cell-surface markers that are specific only for the myeloma cells. Monoclonal antibodies have been developed for some of these myeloma tags and are also in clinical trials, demonstrating that the body's immune system can be harnessed to fight cancer. One of the more exciting examples of such an antibody therapy in myeloma is elotuzumab, which targets a cell-surface glycoprotein and has been shown to induce responses in previously heavily treated patients with relapsed myeloma. Other antibodies have been developed that seek out high-risk features of certain kinds of myeloma, such as the 4:14 translocation, in an attempt to mitigate the added dangers that these mutations can bring. Other small molecule-type drugs are also in development, such as heat-shock protein inhibitors, histone acetylase inhibitors, and cell signal pathway inhibitors, to name a few.

With each new advance made in myeloma, the time free from disease symptoms and overall survival is improved. There have been several key advances in cancer therapy over the last decades, and we are fortunate to have many of these in myeloma. The goal is to one day provide a cure for myeloma and amyloidosis, and there are thousands of doctors and scientists all over the world working on this problem right now. We are all grateful for the support of the especially motivated myeloma community of patients and their families.

It is my sincere hope that Olivia will be able to lead as normal a life as possible, to see her children grow up and her husband, Wai, grow old, together with her.

# LAST WORDS:

Months later, life returned to normal, a new normal. Our family found a routine again, and I reduced my once many volunteering commitments. Our focus was recreating a sense of home: sit down dinners every night, listening to kids talk about their day, and cherishing each other.

Another complication occurred, this time following the insertion of the intercranial stent. The stent was inserted flawlessly by Dr. Patsalides behind my left eye. However, it turns out that one of the prescription drugs that is typically administered after the insertion of a stent can cause blood clots in a very small number of people. I happen to be one of the lucky few! In addition, I was also on Revlimid, which can also cause clotting. I was throwing clots on a fairly regular basis. Some of these traveled to my eyes. After an attempt at surgery from my retinologist, Dr. Chan, where he found clots in the vein and the artery inside my eye, we finally figured out what was happening. Clots. My vision has now mostly returned. After going through the aftermath of the clots, there was a period of calm. Then the pain, my old friend, came back with a vengeance. I was hobbling again, and even used the scooter at times.

*I like to keep my doctors busy.*

Dr. Comenzo and Dr. Mark, puzzled by this outcome, both suggested that the providence of the pain was coming from a source other than multiple myeloma or amyloidosis. So I tried another rheumatologist in Manhattan. On the very first visit, a blood test revealed that in addition to the myeloma, the diabetes, and the amyloidosis, yet another autoimmune disease was present: rheumatoid arthritis! Looking back, it alarms me that both the myeloma and the rheumatoid arthritis were misdiagnosed by local specialists. The irony of it all is that had the local rheumatologist diagnosed me correctly at the very start of this journey, I would never have kept on looking for the source of the pain, and therefore I would never have found the diagnosis of multiple myeloma nor amyloidosis.

It would have been years down the road before they would have been revealed, with possibly dire results.

*All things happen for a reason.*

So about a year after being on Revlimid, we had to stop for fear of more clotting. For the present, I am not on any drugs for multiple myeloma. We are in wait-and-see mode while on blood thinners.

I have no words of wisdom to impart. I have no guidance to give. All I can say is that should you receive a nasty diagnosis, you can cry and wallow in self-pity or you can choose to laugh and hope. Laughter seems to work pretty well for me. I know I didn't start out with a positive outlook—I was more prone to whining about everything before—but the experience of a devastating diagnosis transformed a part of me to something better. I laugh a lot more. I spend time with my family in a meaningful way. I could get smushed by a truck in my car this afternoon, so the realization that my life expectancy is shorter now does not bother me as much. But how I spend the time left is now important. That does not mean I go around hugging my kids all the time, but I try to make our house a welcoming home. I try to make my husband's life a little easier, and I no longer dig big ditches in the backyard to scare him. Having eliminated many of the negative forces in my life has helped improve my outlook immensely. I try to spend a few minutes every day in awe of the magic of the world. And I am thankful to the larger being that made the magic.

*If life hands you limes, make margaritas!*

I go to New York City once a month or more, which is almost a five-hour trip each way. Sometimes I spend nights in hotels, other times I stay with Helene and Dennis and enjoy their company. If I am lucky, I get to break bread with Michael or Eileen. It is no longer an exhausting chore. It can still be exhausting, but it is more pleasant now that I decided to have fun whilst on these trips. Besides seeing several doctors on most visits, I mainly eat well. (What did you expect?) Sometimes I take jaunts to museums, I see some of the sights, and I do a little shopping for my kids. And I spend a lot of time in La Maison du Chocolat.

*Vive le chocolat!*

In addition, the multiple myeloma world is continuing to change and progress, as are the treatments for so many cancers and illnesses. From the time I got the diagnosis of MGUS to now, it is amazing what has transpired in the world of multiple myeloma. Clinical trial drugs then are now routinely prescribed. Drugs that used to have weird names with numbers are now in widespread clinical trials. Newer therapies yet are emerging. Newer combinations of older drugs seem to be effective. One could argue about the pros and cons of drug companies, the cost of these drugs and more, but the end result is that there are better and newer options for us. And more to come.

**And there is hope.**

# Appendix A : Olivia's Post-Transplant Treatment

| Restaurant Name | $ | CC | Décor | Type | Location | Address | Comments |
|---|---|---|---|---|---|---|---|
| 2nd Ave Deli ★ | $$ | Y | OK | Kosher | East Side | 162 E. 33rd St btw Lex & 3rd Ave | My favorite deli! Fantastic hot pastrami, knishes, free pickles & slaw & chocolate soda chaser. |
| Aquamarine | $$ | Y | Good | Asian | East Side | 713 2nd Ave btw 38th & 39th St | Asian fusion & sushi. Lunch specials are good. |
| Banc Café | $$ | Y | Good | Amer | East Side | 431 3rd Ave @ 30th St | Good "in" food, great chocolate molten cake. |
| Ben's Kosher Deli | $$ | Y | Good | Kosher | West Side | 209 W. 38th St btw 7th & 8th Ave | Good hot pastrami, potato pancakes, free pickles & slaw. |
| Big Wong ★ | $ | N | NE | CH | Chinatown | 67 Mott Street btw Canal & Bayard St | Congee, dishes over rice, dirt cheap, noisy, also has full dishes and all roast meats. |
| Boi | $$ | Y | Good | Viet | East Side | 246 E 44 St btw 2nd & 3rd Ave | Pretty place with good food. |
| Cacio e Pepe | $$ | Y | Good | Italian | East Village | 182 2nd Ave btw 11th & 12th St | Get the signature pasta that is made with a wheel of pecorino and black pepper. Then walk to Veniero's for dessert. |
| Café Boulod | $$$ | Y | Good | French | Upper East Side | 20 E 76 St btw 5th & Madison Ave | Fancy dining. A spark is missing. The desserts were excellent. |

| Name | Price | | Rating | Cuisine | Neighborhood | Address | Notes |
|---|---|---|---|---|---|---|---|
| Catham Rest (has red awning, next to Subway) | $ | Y | NE | CH | Chinatown | Catham Square, **CLOSED** | CLOSED! Roast pork buns, big buns, dimsum, dishes over rice, greasy, dirt cheap, noisy. |
| China Fun | $$ | Y | OK | CH | Upper East Side | 1221 2nd Ave @ 64th St | Mediocre stir-fried food, but very good big buns, steamed soup dumplings (six in a bamboo steamer). |
| Daniel's Bagels | $ | | NE | Amer | East Side | 569 3rd Ave btw 37th & 38th St | Good bagels, decent lox and whitefish. |
| El Pote Espanol | $$$ | Y | OK | Span | East Side | 718 2nd Ave btw 38th & 39th St | Spanish, good paella, lobster is popular. |
| Ellen's Stardust Diner | $$ | Y | Good | Amer | Times Square | 1650 Broadway @ 51st St | Singing waitstaff, touristy place. Overpriced, but good burgers and shakes. Just plain fun. |
| Fay Da Bakery / Lunch Box Buffet | $ | | NE | CH | Madison Square Garden | 257 W 34th St, btw 7th & 8th Ave | Fay Da has Chinese baked goods and bubble teas in the front of the store, including roast pork buns. In the back, you get five items for $5. The fried bean curd, pigs feet, and eggplant are good. |
| Havana Central | $$ | Y | Good | Cuban | Times Square | 151 W 46th St btw 6th & 7th Ave | Mojitos happy hour, loud, noisy, stick with pernil, ropa vieja, and flan. Try Margon's across 46 St on the same block. |
| Island Burger | $ | Y | OK | Amer | West Side | 766 9th Ave btw 51st & 52nd St | Great burgers |
| Jing Star | $$ | Y | OK | CH | Chinatown | 27–29 Division Street | Dim sum, dishes over rice, full dishes. |

| Name | Price | | Rating | Type | Area | Address | Notes |
|---|---|---|---|---|---|---|---|
| Joe's Shanghai | $ | Y | OK | CH | Midtown West & Chinatown | 24 West 56th St & 9 Pell St | Soup dumplings! Yum! |
| Juniors | $$ | Y | OK | Amer | Midtown West | 1515 Broadway btw 44th St & 7th Ave & in Grand Central Station | Oh the cheesecake! |
| Kang Suh | $$ | Y | OK | Korean | Koreatown | 1250 Broadway @ 32nd St | Very good with great free starter dishes. |
| Katz's Deli | $$ | | OK | Kosher | Lower East Side | 205 E Houston St btw 1st & Ave A | Corned beef, pastrami, best free pickles, this is the oldest deli in NYC—near Russ & Daughters. |
| Kunjip | $$ | Y | OK | Korean | Koreatown | 9 W. 32nd St btw 5th Ave & Bdwy | Good with good free starter dishes. |
| La Maison du Chocolat ★ | $$$ | Y | Good | Choco | Rockefeller Center | 30 Rockefeller Center, 49th St btw 5th & 6th Ave | Heaven. Must try the guayaquil hot chocolate and the pavé. The macaroons are excellent too. Tearoom on site. |
| Le Cirque | $$$ | Y | Good | French | Midtown East | 151 E 58th St | Luxurious food. Incredible desserts. Spend a fortune but it's worth it, because you get pampered. |
| Lugo Caffe | $$ | Y | Good | Italian | Penn Station | 1 Penn Plaza (33rd St & 8th Ave) | Nice! Salumeria tasting and the pizzas were good. Nice wine selection. |
| Margon | $ | Y | NE | Cuban | Times Square | 136 W 46th St btw 6th & 7th Ave | Pernil, oxtail stew, Cuban sandwich. Deeper than a dive, but food is really good. |

| Name | Price | | Rating | Cuisine | Neighborhood | Address | Notes |
|---|---|---|---|---|---|---|---|
| Matsu Sushi | $$ | Y | OK | Japanese | Upper East Side | 411 E. 70th St btw York & 1st Ave | Good sushi. |
| Minamoto Kitchoan | $ | | Good | Pastry | Rockefeller Center | 608 Fifth Ave, 49th St btw 5th & 6th Ave | Traditional Japanese sweets. Red bean paste and beautiful confections. |
| Momofuku Noodle Bar | $ | Y | Good | Asian | East Village | 163 1st Ave, btw 10th and 11th St | The pork shitake buns are sooo good! |
| Naples 45 | $$ | Y | Good | Italian | Grand Central | 45 St & Grand Central Station (Lex) | Good starters. Skip the entrees but get several appetizers. |
| NY Kom Tang Soot Bul Kal Bi ★ | $$ | Y | OK | Korean | Koreatown | 32 W. 32nd St btw 5th Ave & Bdwy | Go upstairs for Korean BBQ—theirs is done with charcoal braziers rather than gas. |
| Ocean Grill | $$$ | Y | Good | Seafood | Upper West Side | 384 Columbus Ave 78th St btw Columbus & Amsterdam | Fabulous swordfish entrée. Appetizers so-so. |
| Osteria Laguna | $$ | Y | Good | Italian | East Side | 209 E 42nd St btw 2nd & 3rd Ave | Very good from pizza to pastas. Try grilled calamari appetizer. Tiramisu is wow! |
| Phoenix Garden | $$ | N | OK | CH | East Side | 242 E. 40th St btw 2nd & 3rd Ave | Excellent Chinese food, try conch, fried tofu with shrimp paste, steamed fish. |
| Russ & Daughters | $$ | Y | NE | Takeout | Lower East Side | 179 E. Houston St. btw 1st & Ave A | Best smoked fish, lox, caviar, good cream cheese and bagels. This is take-out only. GREAT! |
| Shanghai Mong | $$ | Y | OK | Asian | Koreatown | 30 W. 32nd St btw 5th Ave & Bdwy | Stir-fried Spicy Seafood Noodles. |

| Name | Price | Res | Rating | Cuisine | Neighborhood | Address | Description |
|---|---|---|---|---|---|---|---|
| Smorgas Chef | $$ | | Good | Swedish | Midtown | 58 Park Ave btw 37th & 38th St | Modern setting, weekend brunch. IKEA meets Marrimeko. |
| Stamatis ★ | $$ | Y | Good | Greek | Queens | 29-09 23rd Ave, Astoria (Queens) | Good food with great grilled meats and seafood. |
| Tex Mex Grill | $ | Y | NE | Mex | East Side | 573 2nd Ave near 32nd St | Hole in the wall, dirt cheap, fresh tortillas. |
| Townhouse Diner | $$ | Y | NE | Amer | East Side | 696 2nd Ave btw 37th & 38th St | Decent diner, good souvlaki, plain food. |
| Vanessa's Dumplings | $ | Y | NE | CH | East Village | 220 E. 14th St btw 2nd & 3rd Ave | Five dumplings for $2. |
| Veniero's Pastry ★ | $ | Y | OK | Pastry | East Village | 11 St & 1st Ave | Italian pastry shop: great pastries and coffees. |
| 1Wonjo | $$ | Y | OK | Korean | Koreatown | 23 W. 32nd St btw 5th Ave & Bdwy | Good with good free starter dishes. |
| Wu Liang Ye ★ | $$ | Y | OK | CH | Rockefeller Center | 36 W. 48th St btw 5th & 6th Ave | Good authentic Szechuan food. Belly pork appetizer is fabulous! |
| XO | $ | | NE | CH | Chinatown | 148 Hester St btw Elizabeth & Bowery | Unusual and large selection of snacks and dishes, noisy. |

NE : Nonexistent
Viet: Vietnamese
CH: Chinese
Amer: American
CC: Credit Cards accepted

Places with stars indicate those that provided much joy. All these places contributed to my recovery after the stem cell transplant as well as to my weight gain. Sushi places are underrepresented due to dietary restrictions dictated by the doctors (sigh).

Made in the USA
Lexington, KY
16 April 2013